SPECIAL DIET COOKBOOKS
MULTIPLE SCLEROSIS

To Nancy & Gary

Christmas '93

Love Stan & Sharon

SPECIAL DIET COOKBOOKS

MULTIPLE SCLEROSIS

Healthy menus to help in the management
of multiple sclerosis

Geraldine Fitzgerald and Fenella Briscoe

Published in collaboration with Action for Research into Multiple Sclerosis

THORSONS PUBLISHING GROUP

First published in 1989

British Library Cataloguing in Publication Data

Fitzgerald, Geraldine
  Special diets cookbook: multiple sclerosis
  1. Man. Multiple sclerosis. Therapy.
  Diet
  I. Title   II. Briscoe, Fenella
  616.8'340654

  ISBN 0-7225-1810-2

Photographs on cover are of
Home-made Pizza (*front*, recipe on page 103)
and Cranberry Nut Loaf (*back*, recipe on page
51).

Text illustrations by Juanita Puddifoot

Published by Thorsons Publishers Limited,
Wellingborough, Northamptonshire,
NN8 2RQ, England

Printed in Great Britain by
The Bath Press, Avon

10 9 8 7 6 5 4 3

CONTENTS

INTRODUCTION

The purpose of this book is to demonstrate how easy it can be to follow the healthy eating plan recommended by ARMS (Action for Research into Multiple Sclerosis) for people with multiple sclerosis. Many people see changing their eating pattern as restrictive. However, following these guidelines you will find that there is a wide range of foods available — probably much more varied and interesting than the type of food found in the average British diet.

The menus and recipes contained in this book make up an eating plan that is pleasurable, fun and versatile. They have been devised for anybody who has multiple sclerosis, people who have been recently diagnosed and are finding out about nutrition as part of the self-help approach, but also for those who have been following a diet for many years and feel they need new inspiration.

The ARMS approach to nutrition is designed to provide sound nutritional advice for general health, whilst also ensuring an adequate supply of all the nutrients that support the nervous system. It is suitable — and beneficial — for the whole family, so there is no need to cook separate meals. Emphasis is placed on the fat content of the foods, and the recipes are therefore of interest to anyone wishing to lower the amount of fat in their diet, and to eat more healthily. The ARMS eating plan contains guidelines on foods to include and foods to avoid, see Table 1 (page 8). More detailed information can be found in the booklet 'Why a Diet Rich in Fatty Acids?', available from ARMS (for address see page 14).

We have worked as nutritionists with ARMS for many years, providing nutritional counselling for people with multiple sclerosis, and many people have asked us for examples of what the guidelines mean on a day-to-day basis. Daily menus for a month and new recipes each day help to demonstrate how to put the guidelines into action, and for the special occasion we have given several special menus for dinner parties — one with a British theme, using game, and others with Spanish, Italian, Middle Eastern or Oriental themes, all low in fat, and quite delicious. However, as everybody is an individual, it is advised that before making any changes to your diet you visit a dietitian to get expert advice. This means that you will gain maximum benefit from the eating plan.

Table 1: Diet rich in essential fatty acids ____

Some general rules

1. Use polyunsaturated margarine and oils.
2. Eat at least 3 helpings of fish each week.
3. Eat 225g (½lb) liver each week.
4. Eat a large helping of dark green vegetables daily.
5. Eat some raw vegetables daily, as a salad, with French dressing.
6. Eat some linseeds or 'Linusit Gold' daily.
7. Eat some fresh fruit daily.
8. Eat as much fresh food as possible in preference to processed food.
9. Choose lean cuts of meat, and trim all fat away from meat before cooking.
10. Avoid hard animal fats like butter, lard, suet, dripping, and fatty foods such as cream, hard cheese, etc.
11. Eat wholegrain cereals and wholemeal bread rather than refined cereals.
12. Cut down on sugar and foods containing sugar.

So, why is there an eating plan for MS? ____

There are two reasons for suggesting that people with MS follow a certain eating plan:

1. General good health.
2. As a way of managing MS.

The added bonus is that by becoming more aware of nutrition and what you eat, it is easier to judge whether the advice given to you by friends and family is sound or not. It seems that everyone is an amateur nutritionist!

There is a great deal of scientific evidence suggesting that diet has a role in MS. Studies which looked at the areas of the world where MS occurred found that it was closely linked with the amount of saturated animal fat in the diet. Investigations of the amounts of fat in the blood have shown that some people with MS tend to be low in the polyunsaturated fat known as linoleic acid. Linoleic acid (an essential fatty acid) is found in polyunsaturated oils such as sunflower oil, corn oil, safflower oil and rape seed oil. Scientific trials were carried out in the 1970s in which people with MS were given sunflower oil. It was shown that this reduced the number and severity of relapses. In people who had early MS it was shown to slow down the progression of the disease.

Professor Swank, in the United States, has been advising people to follow a low-fat diet for many years. He finds that by doing so the number of relapses is reduced and the progression of the disease is slowed down. Professor Michael Crawford devised a dietary approach which has been adopted by ARMS. It combines the two previous methods of approach by increasing the amount of all the essential fatty acids (EFAs), and by decreasing the amount of saturated fat. There is also an increase in the vitamins, minerals, trace elements and fibre that the body needs for general health, as well as those that maintain the nervous system. All this is done by eating foods high in nutrients, and avoiding foods that are highly processed and tend to be low in nutrients. A fuller explanation about the fatty acids can be found in the ARMS booklet (see page 14).

Results from the ARMS Nutrition and Exercise Study

A long-term study is being carried out at the ARMS Research Unit, investigating the effects of the diet. Over 500 patients attend the Unit and many take part in research. A nutrition and exercise study is one of the ongoing projects. Nutritional, biochemical, neurological and physiotherapy assessments have been carried out every six months. The results of 83 people who had followed the diet for between three and five years have been analysed. The intake of dietary EFAs correlated with increases in the blood plasma. Analysis of the red blood cells (RBC) of patients revealed abnormally low levels of linoleic acid prior to dietary counselling. After following the diet for six to nine months the RBC membrane fatty acid levels returned to normal values. This implies that abnormalities can be corrected.

The neurological assessment used was the Kurtzke scale. For the group as a whole this did not change over the three-year period. The effect of how closely the guidelines were followed was analysed using a nutrient scoring system. This scored for intakes of key nutrients, including fat intake and associated vitamins, minerals and trace elements. Those scoring above a certain level throughout the three years showed no significant changes on the Kurtzke scale across time. People scoring below 55 per cent on diet showed a significant deterioration. Trends in the relapse data suggested that those complying more closely to the diet had fewer and shorter relapses. Therefore, the more closely the EFA diet was followed, the more beneficial it would appear to be.

Guide to nutritional information

Nutritional information is provided on the menu and recipe pages. Values are given for:

1. The amount of fat per recipe and per day.
2. The ratio of the polyunsaturated fats to saturated fats.
3. The percentage of calories as fat.
4. The amount of fibre.
5. Calories per day.

Menus

The menus have been carefully calculated to meet the ARMS nutritional targets for all nutrients on a weekly basis (see Table 2, page 11). These targets are, in some cases, equivalent to those set by the DHSS, but in some cases they are higher. The nutrients for which an increased intake has been advocated are those involved in the protection and conversion of the fatty acids in the body. For example, the ARMS target for vitamin C is 100–120mg. The UK recommended daily intake set by the DHSS, is 30mg. Vitamin C acts as an antioxidant, which means it protects the polyunsaturated fats from oxidation and turning into saturated fats. As the amount of polyunsaturated fats is being increased, it seems likely that there is an increased need for the associated vitamins, minerals and trace elements, such as vitamin C. So, although the intakes of all the nutrients are not given, all the menus have been calculated to meet these on a weekly basis.

Each recipe has the grams of fat per portion (28g = 1 oz). The aim is to keep the total amount of fat low. This should help you to learn which types of food are high in fat and which are low. The total number of grams of fat per day is given. This is kept to below 75g/day, i.e., less than 3 oz/day of total fat. The ratio of polyunsaturated to saturated fat is called the P/S ratio and is calculated by dividing the amounts of polyunsaturated fat by the saturated fat.

$$\text{P/S ratio} = \frac{\text{g of polyunsaturated fat}}{\text{g of saturated fat}}$$

Table 2: ARMS nutrient target levels

Nutrient	British RDA (Recommended Daily Allowance)	ARMS target
FIBRE (g)	30	above 30
CALORIES *MEN*	2510	2000
WOMEN	1800	1800
VITAMIN C (mg)	30	120
VITAMIN E (mg)	—	12
VITAMIN B_{12} (μg)	3	30
FOLIC ACID (μg)	300	350
VITAMIN B_6 (mg)	2	2
(B_1) THIAMIN (mg) *M*	1.0	1.7
W	0.9	1.5
(B_2) RIBOFLAVIN (mg) *M*	1.6	3.3
W	1.3	3.0
NICOTINIC ACID (mg) *M*	18	25
W	15	23
ZINC (mg)	NO RDA	12
IRON (mg) *M*	10	16
W	12	16
COPPER (mg)	NO RDA	4
CALCIUM (mg)	500	800

The figure quoted for the average British person is a P/S ratio of 0.3:1 showing that the amount of saturated fat in the diet far outweighs the amount of polyunsaturated. This is not thought to be healthy for anyone and a high intake of mainly saturated fats is associated with an increased risk of heart disease. The P/S ratio for the type of food we are recommending is between 1 and 2. Some days it may be over, but the average weekly value will fall in this range (3). The percentage of calories that come from fat is also given. The total amount of fat should be low, with an emphasis on the poly-unsaturates, i.e., P/S above 1. The average British intake of calories from fat is thought to be 40 per cent, the ARMS target is 30 per cent or below.

The amount of fibre per day (4) is given in grams. Fibre is an essential part of any healthy diet, and is found in wholegrain cereals, fruit, vegetables, nuts and legumes. The recommendation is for a minimum of 30g/day. This helps relieve problems such as constipation. If someone has been following a low-fibre diet for many years, it may take a while for the body to adapt to the change, and the increased fibre should be added gradually. Anyone concerned about this should check with a dietitian.

Calorie intake for each day has been calculated (5), including margarine and oil as appropriate and 300ml (½ pint) of skimmed milk per day. Milk can be used freely, unless someone is trying to lose weight, but for every extra 300ml (½ pint) of skimmed milk, add 100Kcals. The calculations have been based on 1700–1800Kcals/day, but everyone has different calorie requirements, depending on how much energy they use throughout the day. Therefore, if you are feeling hungry and losing weight that you don't need to, increase portion sizes, but try to avoid increasing the amount of fat. Conversely, if someone starts to gain weight who should not do so, then portion sizes should be smaller. A GP referral to a dietitian always ensures that alterations made are the best for you. For people who don't need to lose weight, there is no reason why snacks cannot be included, but careful attention should be paid to the type, so as not to increase the fat intake.

Low-fat snacks to include

1. Fresh fruit

2. Dried fruit
3. Slice of wholemeal bread/toast
4. Sunflower seeds/pumpkin seeds
5. Salad — one woman we know keeps a bowl of coleslaw in the fridge to nibble on.
6. Yogurt/fromage frais/cottage cheese
7. Home-made cakes and biscuits, using polyunsaturated fat, but check the total fat for that day.

High-fat snacks to avoid

1. Crisps
2. Chocolate
3. Shop-bought biscuits
4. Shop-bought cakes

Recipes

For each recipe the grams of fat per portion have been given. All recipes serve four people, unless otherwise stated.

Margarines and oils

Throughout the book we have referred to 'suitable' margarines and oils. By this, we mean ones which are high in polyunsaturates. These include sunflower, safflower, corn, soya, rape seed, grape and walnut oils. Never use a blended vegetable oil, as these are mixtures of differing oils and have a higher amount of saturates in them. When buying products, check labels, and if the product contains hydrogenated vegetable fats or oils, try to avoid it. Hydrogenation means that they have become saturated.

Just because the polyunsaturates are good for you, this does *not* mean that spreading margarine thickly and increasing the amount of oil in the recipes is better. Far from it, if this approach is used then it will increase the total fat and P/S ratio above the target level. Therefore, use margarine and oils in normal amounts.

Portion sizes

A result of keeping the fat content of the diet low is that people have to eat more of the less calorie-dense foods. Each gram of fat contains more calories than proteins and carbohydrates. The net result is that to keep the calories at the same level, larger portions may be needed.

We have made our calculations on the basis of the following portion sizes:

Green vegetables — 100-120g (3½-4¼ oz)
Accompanying vegetables — 75g (2¾ oz)
Salads — 100-120g (3½-4¼ oz)
Potatoes, rice, pasta — 150-200g (5¼-7 oz)
Breakfast cereal — 60g (2¼ oz)
Slice of wholemeal bread 50g (1¾ oz)

Again, these may have to be adjusted to suit the individual, but if in doubt, consult a dietitian.

Cooking aids

Some people may have difficulty in the preparation of their food. It is possible to overcome many of these difficulties by the use of specially designed cooking aids or, in some cases, by the adaptation of the kitchen. To see if one can benefit from any of the former, it is advisable to contact the Occupational Therapy department of the social services. They can advise on the appropriate gadgets, and can also recommend the best way to plan a kitchen, or adapt one.

Two organizations which provide further information are The Royal Association for Disability and Rehabilitation (RADAR) and the Disabled Living Foundation (DLF). RADAR,

25 Mortimer Street, London W1N 8AB (Tel: 01-637 5400) provides information and advice in many areas, including access, housing, holidays, mobility and general welfare. The DLF, 380-384 Harrow Road, London W9 2HU (Tel: 01-289 6111) has a comprehensive exhibition of aids, providing a centre for people to try out equipment (an apppointment needs to be made first). It also sends out information on the aids available.

The Gas Boards and Electricity Boards provide free advice about choosing cookers and adapting the controls — contact your local boards to find out about this.

What is ARMS?

In 1974, a group of 30 people — either with MS themselves or closely related to someone with MS — set up the original Multiple Sclerosis Action Group. Because the Group was soon concentrating its efforts on research, in 1975 it was renamed Action for Research into Multiple Sclerosis. ARMS is a registered charity with a membership of over 7000, which raises £½ million a year to provide its own voluntary funding.

ARMS looks into the cause, diagnosis, treatment, cure and prevention of MS. It seeks to educate the public, patients and professionals about the disease by publishing:

Research papers (ARMS Education Service)
Authoritative articles
A regular magazine, ARMS LINK, informing members on all aspects of the disease, and making available ideas for better disease management.

ARMS offers individuals:
Therapy advice based on scientific studies.
Membership of a network of therapy groups.
A 24-hour telephone counselling service.
Information resources open to professionals and patients alike.

For further information contact:

ARMS,
4A Chapel Hill,
Stansted,
Essex, CM23 8AG
(Tel: 0279 815553)

RECIPES
AND MENUS

WEEK 1

Sunday

Half grapefruit
Muesli
Skimmed milk
Wholemeal toast
Marmalade

Roast beef (lean)
Jacket potato
Gravy
Broccoli
Sweetcorn
Orange Mousse (page 18)
Muesli Chews (see Week 1, Thursday, page 32)

Savoury Rice Salad (page 18)
Wholemeal bread
Fresh fruit

Nutritional Information:

Fat (gms)	42
P/S ratio	1.68
Fat (%)	23
Fibre (gms)	34
Energy (Kcals)	1700

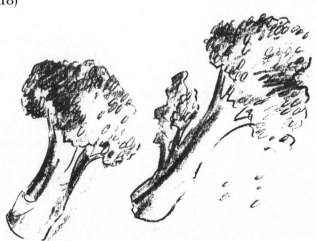

Orange Mousse

A variety of low-fat soft cheeses are available and can be used in many different recipes, including the preparation of quick desserts such as this one. Suitable varieties to use are quark, fromage frais, cottage cheese (though this does not have the smooth texture of the others) and Ricotta, an Italian soft cheese.

Fat per portion = 2g

15g (½ oz) powdered gelatine
2 tablespoons hot water
225g (8 oz) skimmed milk soft cheese
170ml (6 fl oz) can frozen orange juice, thawed
2 egg whites

1. Sprinkle the gelatine over the hot water in a cup and stir until dissolved.
2. Whisk the soft cheese, add the orange juice and gelatine mixture.
3. Whisk the egg whites until stiff and fold into the orange mixture.
4. Pour into serving glasses and chill until set.

Savoury Rice Salad

Salads are quick meals to make, as well as being good for you, rich in vitamins, minerals and fibre. The addition of wholemeal pasta or brown rice to a salad makes a satisfying main meal, served with some crusty wholemeal bread.

Fat per portion = 13g

455g (1 lb) brown rice
1 bunch of spring onions, chopped
2 green peppers, cored, de-seeded and sliced
1 red pepper, cored, de-seeded and sliced
2 celery stalks, chopped
2 small carrots, grated
85g (3 oz) cashew nuts
28g (1 oz) sunflower seeds
Freshly ground black pepper
4 tablespoons of dressing from the selection on page 123

1. Cook the brown rice in boiling water until tender (about 40 minutes).
2. Drain the rice, rinse in cold water and drain well again.
3. Add the spring onions, green peppers, red pepper, celery, carrots, nuts and sunflower seeds.
4. Season with the pepper and toss in the dressing of your choice.
5. Chill in the refrigerator until required.

Monday

Orange juice
Apple Oatmeal (page 20)
Skimmed milk
Wholemeal toast
Sunflower seed spread

Plaice with lemon
Boiled potatoes
Peas
Kale
Apricot Tart (page 20)

Lentil Pâté sandwiches (page 21)
Side salad with dressing
Fresh fruit/yogurt

Nutritional Information:

Fat (gms)	34
P/S ratio	2.8
Fat (%)	17
Fibre (gms)	55
Energy (Kcals)	1900

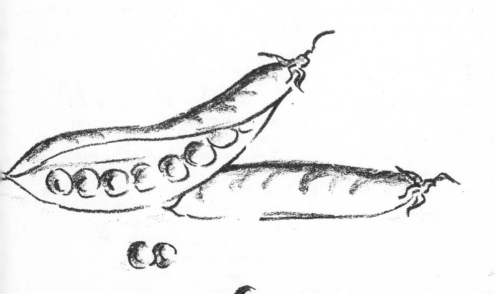

Apple Oatmeal

Serves 2

Fresh or dried fruit can be added to any breakfast cereal to give variety, and to increase the fibre and vitamins in the diet.

Fat per portion = 3g if served with 100ml skimmed milk
Fat per portion = 4g if served with 100ml yogurt

1 cup rolled oats
2 cups cold water
2 apples, chopped
1 teaspoon ground nutmeg or cinnamon

1. Cook rolled oats in the water for about 10 minutes on a low heat.
2. Add the chopped apples and spice and continue cooking for a further 5 minutes, or until the apples are cooked to your taste.
3. Serve with yogurt or skimmed milk.

Apricot Tart

This makes use of store-cupboard items and, since it uses breadcrumbs instead of pastry and skimmed milk in the custard, it is a low-fat sweet.

Fat per portion = 1g

Large tin (411g/14½ oz) of apricots, in natural juice
55g (2 oz) wholemeal breadcrumbs
1 egg white
1 tablespoon sugar
1 tablespoon skimmed milk powder
1 tablespoon custard powder
285ml (½ pint) skimmed milk

1. Drain the fruit, reserving the juice.
2. Put the breadcrumbs into an ovenproof dish and moisten with as much of the juice as necessary.
3. Arrange the apricots on the crumb base.
4. Whisk together the egg white, sugar, milk powder and custard powder.
5. Gradually add the liquid milk to the egg white mixture, then pour carefully over the apricots.
6. Bake at 400°F (200°C/Gas Mark 4) until the custard is set (about 1 hour).
7. Serve cold.

Lentil Pâté

Serves 4–6

Lentils, like all pulses, are a good source of the essential fatty acids and are also high in fibre.

Fat per portion = 4g

115g (4 oz) lentils
2 tablespoons suitable oil
1 small onion, finely chopped
1 clove garlic, crushed
55g (2 oz) mushrooms, sliced (optional)
1 tablespoon tomato purée
1 tablespoon chopped parsley
Freshly ground black pepper

1. Soak the lentils for an hour or so, or overnight. Drain and rinse, then add just under 285ml (½ pint) of water. Bring to the boil and then simmer for 20 minutes until the lentils are very tender.
2. Drain off any extra liquid.
3. Heat the oil. Fry the onion and garlic. Add the mushrooms and continue to cook until they are just soft.
4. Remove from the heat and mix in the lentils, tomato purée and parsley. Add black pepper, to taste.
5. Chill before using.

Tuesday

Grapefruit juice
Baked beans
Wholemeal toast

Liver with Orange (page 23) garnished with
    watercress
Wholewheat noodles
Green beans
Grilled tomatoes
Strawberry Fluff (page 24)

Tuna with jacket potato with Yogurt Dressing
    (page 24)
Side salad
Fruit

Nutritional Information:

Fat (gms)	56
P/S ratio	1.7
Fat (%)	29
Fibre (gms)	48
Energy (Kcals)	1700

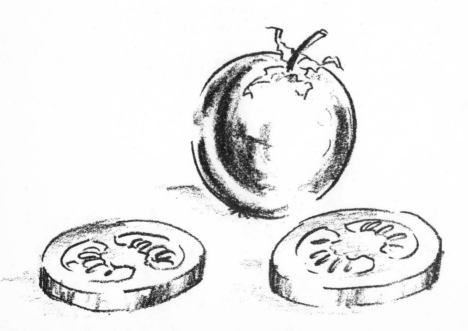

Liver with Orange

Liver is a lean source of high quality protein, also providing vitamins A and B and iron. It is particularly important for you as a source of arachidonic acid, one of the essential fatty acids.

Fat per portion = 18g

2 tablespoons suitable oil
2 medium onions, sliced
4 slices lamb's or pig's liver
2 tablespoons wholemeal flour, seasoned with black pepper and mixed herbs (optional)
4 tablespoons orange juice
1 tablespoon soya sauce
2 oranges, sliced

1. Heat the oil in a frying pan. Add the onions and fry until transparent.
2. Coat the liver with the flour.
3. Fry the liver gently for 3–4 minutes on each side. Add the orange juice, soya sauce and orange slices, then cook for a further 2–3 minutes.
4. If you prefer extra sauce, add more orange juice and thicken with cornflour.

Strawberry Fluff

Serves 6

This recipe enables you to make a mousse from low-fat ingredients. Any fruit can be substituted for the strawberries, using the appropriately-flavoured jelly.

Fat per portion = 9g

55g (2 oz) suitable margarine
115g (4 oz) digestive biscuits, crushed
1 packet strawberry jelly
140ml (¼ pint) boiling water
225g (8 oz) skimmed milk soft cheese
225g (8 oz) natural yogurt
Strawberries, to decorate

1. Melt the margarine in a saucepan over a low heat, and add the crushed biscuits. Mix well and press into a 18cm (7-inch) loose-bottomed round cake tin.
2. Dissolve the jelly in the boiling water. Allow to cool, but not to set.
3. Beat the soft cheese, yogurt and jelly together until smooth.
4. Pour the mixture over the cooled base in the tin and leave to set in the fridge. Turn out and decorate with fruit before serving.

Yogurt Dressing

This is a particularly useful dressing for jacket potatoes or a salad. It is enough for several days and can be stored successfully in the fridge.

Fat per portion is negligible.

285ml (½ pint) natural yogurt
4 tablespoons lemon juice
½ teaspoon dry mustard
1 clove garlic, crushed
1 teaspoon paprika

Mix all the ingredients together thoroughly, then chill.

Wednesday

Orange juice
Wholegrain cereal
Sultanas/fresh fruit
Wholemeal toast
Sesame seed spread

Pandy's Chick Peas (page 26)
Stir-fried Vegetables (page 27)
Brown rice
Apple Crunch (page 27)

Mackerel pâté sandwiches
Hot spiced fruit salad

Nutritional Information:

Fat (gms)	48
P/S ratio	2.7
Fat (%)	24
Fibre (gms)	33
Energy (Kcals)	1800

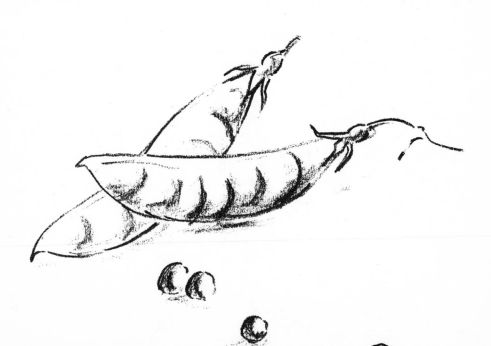

Pandy's Chick Peas

Fat per portion = 15g

2 medium onions
2 cloves garlic
4 tablespoons suitable oil
2 teaspoons cumin seeds
2 teaspoons ground coriander
1 teaspoon ground turmeric
2 teaspoons ground paprika
½ teaspoon cayenne pepper
225g (½ lb) chick peas, cooked until soft
  (reserve 140ml (¼ pint) cooking liquid)
1 tablespoon tomato purée
2 tablespoons chopped mint
140ml (¼ pint) natural yogurt

1. Finely chop onions and garlic.
2. Heat the oil in a saucepan, over a low heat.
3. Stir in the onions, garlic and all the spices and cook until the onions are soft.
4. Stir in the cooked chick peas and tomato purée.
5. Pour in the reserved cooking liquid from the chick peas and bring to the boil.
6. Cover and simmer for 30 minutes.
7. Serve with the chopped mint sprinkled over the top, accompanied by a side bowl of yogurt.

Stir-fried Vegetables

The Chinese method of stir-frying is an ideal way to cook vegetables, as it preserves many of the natural vitamins and minerals which are usually lost in the vegetable water. The vegetables should be cooked for a very short time and remain crisp and tasy. Any selection of vegetables can be used — experiment until you find your own favourite combination.

Fat per portion = 8g

2 tablespoons suitable oil
1 green pepper, pith and seeds removed, cut into strips
1 large onion, sliced in rings
1 clove garlic, crushed
115g (4 oz) carrots, thinly sliced
1 small cauliflower, cut into small florets
115g (4 oz) beansprouts
Seasoning to taste

1. Heat the oil in a wok or large frying pan on a high heat.
2. Put in all the vegetables except the beansprouts and stir-fry for 2 minutes.
3. Add the beansprouts and stir-fry for 1 minute more.
4. Add any desired seasoning, e.g., black pepper, soya sauce, Worcester sauce, and perhaps a dash of sherry or brandy for special occasions.
5. Serve immediately.

Apple Crunch

Breakfast cereals are useful ingredients for quick pudding recipes, and also make useful snacks when eaten with skimmed milk or natural fruit juice.

Fat per portion = 7g

455g (1 lb) cooking apples
2 tablespoons honey
2 tablespoons lemon juice
2 tablespoons brown sugar
55g (2 oz) walnut pieces
55g (2 oz) Shreddies, or similar breakfast cereal

1. Peel, core and slice the apples then cook until tender.
2. Divide between four individual dessert bowls.
3. Place honey, lemon juice and sugar in a small saucepan and heat gently.
4. Add walnuts and crushed cereal to honey mixture, mix well then sprinkle over the apple. Serve hot or cold.

Thursday

Orange juice
Hot Spiced Fruit Salad (page 29), chopped
  nuts and yogurt
Wholemeal toast
Jam or marmalade

Baked Herrings with Mushroom Stuffing
  (page 30)
New potatoes
Salad
Fresh fruit with fromage frais

Spinach and Watercress Soup (page 31)
Wholemeal bread
Muesli Chews (page 32)

Nutritional Information:

Fat (gms)	55
P/S ratio	2.0
Fat (%)	29
Fibre (gms)	28
Energy (Kcals)	1700

Hot Spiced Fruit Salad

Using a wide-mouthed vacuum flask is ideal for someone who is unable to prepare food themselves, and who has to have food prepared for them before it is actually required. A flask of this kind may also be useful to keep warm such things as Chilli con Carne (Friday, Week 2, page 56).

Fat per portion is negligible.

225g (8 oz) dried fruit salad, or a mixture of dried apricots, peaches, apple rings, pears prunes, raisins or sultanas

570ml (1 pint) pure fruit juice, e.g. apple juice

½ teaspoon ground cinnamon

1. Place the dried fruits, juice and cinnamon in a bowl and leave to soak overnight.
2. Transfer to a saucepan and bring to the boil, then simmer for 10–15 minutes.
3. Either serve immediately, or tip into a wide-mouthed vacuum flask with enough liquid to cover by 2.5cm (1 inch) and cover until it is wanted.

Baked Herrings with Mushroom Stuffing

Oily fish, such as herrings or mackerel, are not only an important part of your diet but they are also economical and very convenient. So many flavours can be added to the fish during cooking, either by stuffing the fish — as here — or by making slashes at 2.5cm (1 inch) intervals through the skin of the fish and seasoning from the outside through these.

Fat per portion = 19g

4 large herrings

Stuffing:

55g (2 oz) mushrooms, chopped finely
1 teaspoon suitable oil
115g (4 oz) fresh wholemeal breadcrumbs, softened in skimmed milk, then squeezed
Clove garlic, crushed
1 teaspoon marjoram
Pinch oregano
1 egg
Salt and pepper

1. Clean the herrings. Remove the heads and tails and open out.
2. Fry the mushrooms in the oil and transfer to a dish. Mix all the other stuffing ingredients and add to the mushrooms.
3. Stuff the herrings with this mixture, then close them up.
4. Place in an oven-proof dish, cover with foil and bake in a moderate oven for 30 minutes.

Spinach and Watercress Soup

Serves 4–6

A different way to include a dark green leafy vegetable in your diet, although it is important to eat some leafy vegetables raw whenever possible, as they are a rich source of iron and folic acid.

Fat per portion = 6g

115g (4 oz) spinach
1 bunch watercress
28g (1 oz) suitable margarine
1 medium onion, chopped
1 large potato
570ml (1 pint) chicken stock
285ml (½ pint) skimmed milk
Seasoning, to taste

1. Wash the watercress and spinach, remove the coarse stalks and chop the remainder.
2. Melt the margarine and fry the onion until soft.
3. Peel the potato and cut into large dice.
4. Add the potato, chopped spinach and watercress to the pan and toss with onion and butter.
5. Allow to cook for 1 minute, then add stock and skimmed milk.
6. Bring to the boil, cover and simmer for 30 minutes.
7. Remove from the heat and purée the soup.
8. Return to the pan, reheat, season and serve.

Muesli Chews

Makes 16

Made from store-cupboard items, these are quick and easy and invaluable to have in the cupboard for a nourishing snack. They are also nice to serve with fresh fruit or mousse (see Sunday, Week 1, page 17).

Fat per chew = 5g

85g (3 oz) suitable margarine
115g (4 oz) demerara sugar
2 tablespoons honey
1 medium banana, peeled and mashed
28g (1 oz) sultanas
285g (10 oz) muesli

1. Set the oven to moderate, 350°F (180°C/Gas Mark 4).
2. Cream the margarine until soft, then beat in the sugar, honey and banana.
3. Stir in the sultanas and muesli.
4. Spoon into a greased 18×28cm (7×11 inch) Swiss roll tin and spread the mixture level.
5. Bake towards the top of the oven for 25–30 minutes.
6. Cut into fingers in the tin while still warm.
7. Leave to become quite cold before removing from the tin and separating the fingers.

Friday

Grapefruit juice
Grilled tomatoes and mushrooms on
  wholemeal toast
Wholemeal toast with marmalade

Roast chicken
Jacket potatoes
Spinach
Carrots
Gravy
Quick Fruit Crumble (page 34) with
  custard

Meat Loaf (page 34)
4 Bean Salad (page 35)
Fruit yogurt

Nutritional Information:

Fat (gms)	51
P/S ratio	1.6
Fat (%)	28
Fibre (gms)	37
Energy (Kcals)	1600

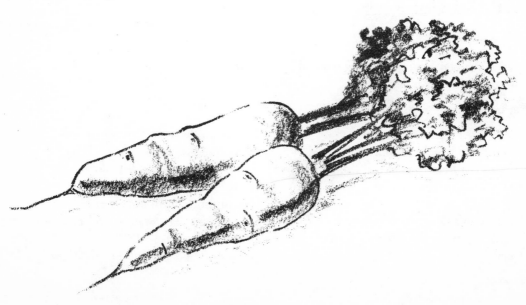

Quick Fruit Crumble

Serves 6

This crumble is quick and easy to make. Leave plenty of juice with the stewed fruit so the mixture is not too dry. The oil sprinkled over the top before baking gives the crumble a really crunchy texture. When you make up an ordinary crumble you can always mix in a little muesli with the crumble mixture to give it a crunchier texture.

Fat per portion = 10g

455g (1 lb) stewed fruit
Muesli (bought, or home-made — see
  Week 3, page 74)
4 tablespoons suitable oil

1. Place the stewed fruit in an oven-proof bowl.
2. Sprinkle the muesli on top of the fruit.
3. Drip the oil over the surface of the muesli.
4. Bake at 350°F (180°C/Gas Mark 4) for 20–25 minutes.
5. Serve hot or cold.

Meat Loaf

Serves 6

This is a super way of including some liver in your diet, and any left over can be used as a savoury sandwich filling.

Fat per portion = 9g

225g (8 oz) pig's liver, minced
225g (8 oz) lean beef, minced
115g (4 oz) fresh wholemeal breadcrumbs
1 tablespoon mixed herbs
½ teaspoon pepper
1 teaspoon salt
4 tablespoons dry cider
1 egg

1. Mix all the ingredients together very thoroughly.
2. Press the mixture very firmly into a 455g (1 lb) loaf tin.
3. Stand the tin in a dish of hot water in the centre of the oven and bake for 1½ hours at 350°F (180°C/Gas Mark 4).
4. Leave to cool in the tin, then chill.

4 Bean Salad

Serves 6–8

Fat per portion = 5g

115g (4 oz) butter beans
115g (4 oz) red kidney beans
115g (4 oz) haricot beans
115g (4 oz) French beans, cut into 2.5cm
   (1 inch) lengths
6 spring onions, chopped
4 tablespoons home-made French dressing
2 tablespoons chopped parsley

1. Soak the butter, kidney and haricot
   beans separately overnight.
2. Drain and place in separate pans, cover
   with cold water, bring to the boil and
   boil steadily for 15 minutes. Lower the
   heat, cover and simmer for 1–1½ hours.
   Drain.
3. Cook the French beans in the usual way,
   then drain.
4. Place all the beans in a serving bowl
   and mix in the onions and dressing
   while the beans are still warm.
5. Leave to cool, then refrigerate for at least
   an hour.
6. Stir in the parsley just before serving.

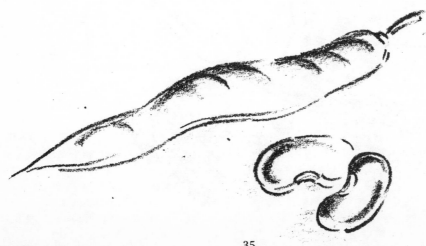

Saturday

Orange juice
Wholegrain cereal and dried fruit
Skimmed milk *or* yogurt
Wholemeal toast
Sunflower spread

Fisherman's Pie (page 37)
Broccoli
Sweetcorn
Apricot and Date Brûlée (page 38)

Chicken and salad sandwiches
Fresh fruit and yogurt

Nutritional Information:

Fat (gms)	36
P/S ratio	1.8
Fat (%)	19
Fibre (gms)	58
Energy (Kcals)	1700

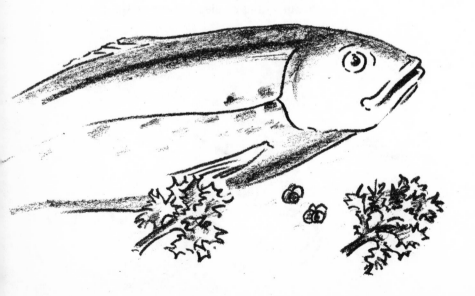

Fisherman's Pie

This tasty fish pie is ideal for serving on many occasions. It freezes well, so it is perfect for batch cooking when you have the time and energy.

Fat per portion = 14g

680g (1½ lbs) white fish
570ml (1 pint) skimmed milk
55g (2 oz) suitable margarine
55g (2 oz) wholemeal flour
Black pepper
115g (4 oz) prawns
3 tablespoons parsley, chopped
1 tablespoon lemon juice
900 (2 lbs) cooked potatoes

1. Put the fish in an oven-proof dish with 140ml (¼ pint) milk. Bake in a hot oven for 15–20 minutes. Strain, reserve the liquid and skin the fish.
2. Melt 45g (1½ oz) margarine in a pan, stir in the flour and cook for 1 minute.
3. Gradually add the milk in which the fish was cooked, then the remainder of the milk, stirring to avoid any lumps forming.
4. Season the sauce, then add the cooked fish, prawns, parsley and lemon juice. Mash the potatoes with the remaining margarine.
5. Pour into a well-greased oven-proof dish and cover with the mashed potatoes. Bake for a further 20 minutes at 400°F (200°C/Gas Mark 6).

Apricot and Date Brûlée

This is a really quick dessert that everyone will love. Any dried fruit of your choice can be substituted for the apricots and dates.

Fat per portion is negligible.

225g (8 oz) plump dried apricots, chopped
225g (8 oz) dates, chopped
4 tablespoons orange juice
140ml (5 fl oz) fromage frais
2 tablespoons demerara sugar

1. Place the apricots and dates in a saucepan with the orange juice. Bring to the boil, cover and simmer for 2 minutes.
2. Pre-heat the grill. Meanwhile, fill four small heatproof ramekin dishes with the fruit mixture, cover each with fromage frais then sprinkle the sugar over.
3. Place the ramekins under the hot grill until the sugar bubbles and turns slightly darker in colour.
4. Remove from under the heat and leave to stand for a minute, until the sugar hardens.

WEEK 2

Sunday

Pineapple juice
Kipper
Wholemeal bread

Portuguese Pork Casserole (page 40)
Spinach
Jacket potato
Figs with Walnuts (page 40)

Middle Eastern Lentil Soup (page 41)
Wholemeal bread
Fruit fromage frais

Nutritional Information:	
Fat (gms)	61
P/S ratio	1.7
Fat (%)	28
Fibre (gms)	42
Energy (Kcals)	1900

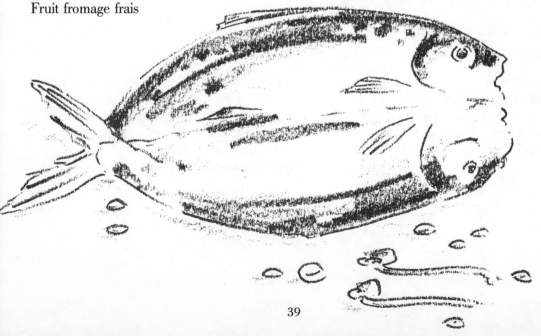

Portuguese Pork Casserole

Fat per portion = 11g

455g (1 lb) pork fillet or shoulder
1 tablespoon suitable oil
1 large onion, sliced thinly
2 cloves garlic, crushed
395 g (14 oz) tin tomatoes
2 carrots, diced
Seasoning to taste
Chicken stock cube (optional)
395g (14 oz) tin chick peas
225g (8 oz) green beans, sliced

1. Trim the fat off the meat and dice into large pieces.
2. Fry the meat in the oil over a high heat to seal.
3. Lower the heat; add the onion, garlic, tomatoes, carrots and seasoning and stock cube if desired.
4. Leave to simmer 1–1½ hours.
5. Drain the chick peas; add the green beans and chick peas to the casserole.
6. Heat for a further 20 minutes to warm through.
7. Serve on a bed of rice or couscous.

Figs with Walnuts

This is a Spanish recipe, but traditionally the figs would be stuffed with the walnuts.

Fat per portion = 5g

20 dried figs
285ml (½ pint) pure orange juice
55g (2 oz) walnuts, chopped finely
Greek yogurt (optional)
Sunflower seeds (optional)

1. Stew the figs in the orange juice for about 15 minutes, until plumped.
2. Sprinkle the walnuts over the figs.
3. Serve with 1 dessertspoon of Greek yogurt on top, if liked.
4. Sprinkle with sunflower seeds if desired.

Middle Eastern Lentil Soup

This soup can be refrigerated and reheated, but as it thickens on cooling it will require a little additional water before reheating.

Fat per portion = 8g

1 onion
2-3 carrots
2 tablespoons sunflower oil
225g (8 oz) yellow lentils
2 chicken/vegetable stockcubes
850ml (1½ pints) water
2 teaspoons cumin spice
1-2 cloves crushed garlic (optional)
A little more sunflower oil
Salt and pepper

1. Chop the onion and carrots and fry in the oil.
2. Rinse the lentils under cold running water.
3. When the onion is transparent, add the lentils, stirring well, over a low heat.
4. Dissolve the stockcubes in the water and after a few minutes add to the vegetables.
5. Bring to the boil then allow to simmer for about 1 hour.
6. If desired, blend the soup and return it to the heat. Keep it warm on a low heat.
7. Meanwhile fry the cumin and crushed garlic on a low heat in very little oil. When golden brown add to the soup and stir well. Season to taste.

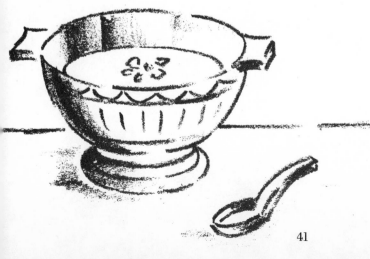

Monday

Grapefruit segments
Grapenuts and skimmed milk
Wholemeal toast
Sunflower seed spread

Liver Italian-style (page 43)
Jacket potato
Beans
Sweetcorn
Fresh fruit yogurt

Cottage cheese
Salad and dressing
Bread roll
Banana Loaf (page 44)

Nutritional Information:

Fat (gms)	52
P/S ratio	1.2
Fat (%)	28
Fibre (gms)	32
Energy (Kcals)	1700

Liver Italian-style

Liver is a lean source of high-quality protein, also providing vitamins A and B, zinc, iron and folic acid. It is particularly important for you as a source of arachidonic acid, one of the essential fatty acids.

Fat per portion = 23g

55g (2 oz) suitable margarine
1 medium onion
115g (4 oz) mushrooms
455g (1 lb) lamb's liver
395g (14 oz) tin tomatoes
1 tablespoon tomato purée
120 ml (4 fl oz) stock
½ teaspoon thyme
½ teaspoon basil
1 bay leaf

1. Melt 28g (1 oz) margarine and fry the onion for 3–5 minutes until soft.
2. Add the mushrooms. Transfer to a casserole.
3. Add the remaining margarine and cook the liver. Transfer to the casserole.
4. Add the tomatoes, purée and stock to the pan. Bring the liquid to the boil. Stir in the seasoning. Cook for 1 minute.
5. Pour over the liver in the casserole. Mix.
6. Bake 30–45 minutes, 350°F (180°C/Gas Mark 4) or until the liver is tender.

Banana Loaf

A really simple quick recipe, suitable for anyone with a liquidizer and especially for those who are unable to spend a long time cooking.

Fat per slice = 5g

1 ripe banana
1 egg
85g (3 oz) sugar
55g (2 oz) suitable margarine
½ teaspoon vanilla essence
½ teaspoon salt
140g (5 oz) wholemeal self-raising flour
½ teaspoon bicarbonate of soda

1. Put the banana, egg, sugar, margarine, vanilla and salt in the liquidizer and blend on maximum speed for 1 minute.
2. Sift the flour and bicarbonate of soda into a bowl and pour the liquidized mixture over.
3. Mix on a low speed just long enough to mix the ingredients thoroughly.
4. Bake in a loaf tin for approximately 45 minutes at 375°F (190°C/Gas Mark 5).

Tuesday

Porridge with skimmed milk
Fresh fruit
Wholemeal toast
Marmalade

Mackerel Kebabs (page 46)
Savoury brown rice
Green salad
Banana Muesli Layer (page 47)

Butterbean and Tomato Soup (page 47)
Wholemeal roll
Yogurt/fresh fruit

Nutritional Information:

Fat (gms)	63
P/S ratio	1.5
Fat (%)	32
Fibre (gms)	33
Energy (Kcals)	1800

Mackerel Kebabs

An unusual way of serving mackerel, useful also for barbecues in the summer. The kebabs are quite 'fiddly' to prepare, so not suitable for anyone who finds hand co-ordination difficult. Although the fat content is quite high, it is mainly due to the oil from the fish, which contains essential fatty acids.

Fat per portion = 29g

4 mackerel, cleaned, gutted and with backbones removed
6 baby onions
4 small tomatoes
4 button mushrooms, wiped clean
1 large green pepper, white pith removed, seeded and cut into 2.5cm (1 inch) wide strips
60ml (2 fl oz) white wine vinegar
60ml (2 fl oz) suitable oil
½ teaspoon salt
½ teaspoon black pepper
1 teaspoon dried oregano

1. Cut each mackerel into 4 or 5 slices.
2. Thread the slices of fish on to skewers alternating with the onions, tomatoes, mushrooms and green pepper strips.
3. In a large shallow dish, combine the vinegar, oil, salt, pepper and oregano.
4. Lay the prepared skewers in the dish and leave to marinate at room temperature for about 2 hours, turning occasionally.
5. Preheat the grill to HIGH.
6. Remove the kebabs from the marinade and place them under the grill.
7. Cook for 8–10 minutes, basting the kebabs with the marinade and turning them frequently, or until the fish flakes easily when tested with a fork.
8. Serve the kebabs immediately on a warmed serving dish.

Banana Muesli Layer

What dessert could be quicker than this!

Fat per portion = 1g

3 bananas
425ml (15 fl oz) natural yogurt
1 tablespoon lemon juice
3 tablespoons clear honey
85g (3 oz) muesli-type breakfast cereal

1. Finely mash the bananas with a fork.
2. Add the yogurt and lemon juice and stir well.
3. Divide between 4 individual glass dishes.
4. Heat the honey in a small pan and stir in the cereal.
5. Sprinkle over the banana mixture.

Butterbean and Tomato Soup

If you forget to soak the beans overnight, use tinned beans instead, but use less salt in the recipe.

Fat per portion is negligible.

225g (8 oz) butterbeans
Bay leaf
850ml (1½ pints) water
395g (14 oz) tin tomatoes
Sliced lemon
Salt to taste
Onion, chopped

1. Soak the butterbeans overnight.
2. Next day simmer all the ingredients until soft.
3. Remove the bay leaf and lemon.
4. Liquidize and season, to taste.

Wednesday

Orange juice
Baked beans on wholemeal toast
Fruit

Lapin à la Moutarde (page 49)
Jacket potato
Broccoli
Carrots
Baked apples and custard (made with
    skimmed milk)

Sandwiches with Hummus (page 50) and
    salad
Cranberry Nut Loaf (page 51)

Nutritional Information:

Fat (gms)	51
P/S ratio	2.5
Fat (%)	21
Fibre (gms)	65
Energy (Kcals)	2100

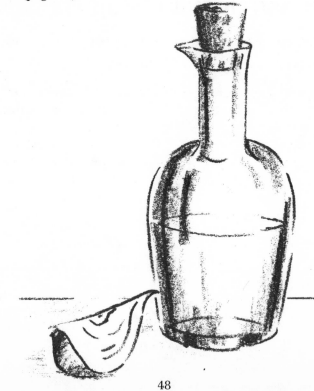

Lapin à la Moutarde
(Rabbit with Mustard Sauce)

Rabbit, like other game meats, is very low in fat but rich in Arachidonic acid.

Fat per portion = 9g

4 rabbit pieces
1 tablespoon vinegar
28g (1 oz) suitable margarine
2 onions, chopped
28g (1 oz) flour
425ml (¾ pint) chicken stock
Salt and pepper
Bouquet garni
2 tablespoons French mustard
Parsley to garnish

1. Soak the rabbit overnight in water, adding the vinegar.
2. Drain and pat dry.
3. Melt the margarine, add the rabbit pieces and onions and cook until brown.
4. Remove and sprinkle in the flour and cook for 2 minutes, stirring.
5. Gradually stir in the stock, bring to the boil, add the salt and pepper and bouquet garni.
6. Place the rabbit and onion mixture in a casserole dish, cover and cook at 350°F (180°C/Gas Mark 4) for about 1½ hours, or until the rabbit is tender.
7. Remove the bouquet garni, stir in the mustard and serve sprinkled with parsley.

Hummus

Hummus is delicious with warm wholemeal pitta bread. Tahini is a strong nutty paste made from crushed sesame seeds which are rich in calcium and provide essential fatty acids.

Fat per portion = 8g

115g (4 oz) dried chick peas
1-2 cloves garlic, crushed
2 tablespoons lemon juice
4 teaspoons suitable oil
Sea salt
2 teaspoons tahini

To garnish:

Paprika, lemon wedges, cucumber, olives

1. Soak, drain and rinse the chick peas then cook for about an hour until tender and drain, preserving the liquid.
2. Liquidize or mash the chick peas with 4-5 teaspoons of the cooking liquid, garlic, lemon juice, and half the oil. Thin if necessary with more cooking liquid.
3. Season and chill.
4. Serve spread on a flat dish, trickle tahini around the edge. Dribble remaining oil over, sprinkle with paprika and garnish as desired.

Cranberry Nut Loaf

A lovely moist loaf. Use frozen or tinned cranberries so that you can make it any time of the year. Sunflower seeds could also be added if you wish.

Fat per slice = 9g

225g (8 oz) plain wholemeal flour
1½ teaspoons baking powder
½ teaspoon bicarbonate of soda
1 teaspoon salt
55g (2 oz) suitable margarine
170g (6 oz) sugar
140ml (¼ pint) orange juice
1 tablespoon grated orange rind
1 egg, beaten
85g (3 oz) chopped walnuts
115g (4 oz) chopped cranberries

1. Grease and line a 455g (1 lb) loaf tin.
2. Sift together the flour, baking powder, bicarbonate of soda and salt. Rub in the margarine and add the sugar.
3. Mix the orange juice, rind and egg.
4. Pour the orange juice mixture on to the dry ingredients and mix lightly.
5. Fold in the walnuts and cranberries.
6. Turn into the tin and bake in the centre of the oven at 350°F (180°C/Gas Mark 4) for 1-1¼ hours.

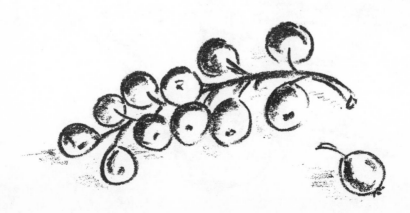

Thursday

Grapefruit segments
Bran cereal
Skimmed milk
Wholemeal toast
Marmalade

Boston Braised Cod (page 53)
Spinach
Leeks
Summer Fruits Pudding (page 54) with
   yogurt

Jacket potato with cottage cheese
Rice salad with dressing
Fresh fruit

Nutritional Information:

Fat (gms)	46
P/S ratio	1.8
Fat (%)	25
Fibre (gms)	60
Energy (Kcals)	1700

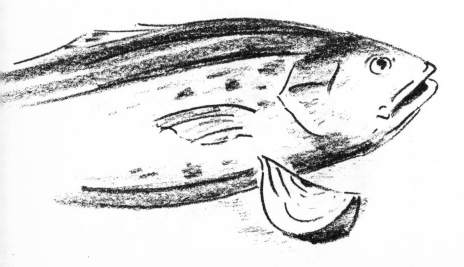

Boston Braised Cod

Serves 2

This recipe shows how meat or fish can be cooked together with vegetables in one pan to be labour-saving. A multi-cooker is particularly suitable for this form of cooking. This recipe can be made to serve 1 portion, using a 200g (7 oz) tin of beans and reducing the other ingredients by half.

Fat per portion = 16g

2 tablespoons oil
2 medium potatoes
1 medium onion, sliced
2 frozen cod steaks
1 teaspoon vinegar
1 teaspoon brown sugar
Salt and pepper
395g (14 oz) tin baked beans

1. Put the oil in a non-stick shallow pan (preferably a frying pan) with a lid.
2. Thinly slice the potatoes and add to the oil, with the onion.
3. Stir gently, cover and cook over moderate heat for about 5 minutes, until the vegetables begin to soften.
4. Press the cod steaks into the bed of vegetables.
5. Sprinkle over the vinegar and sugar and season lightly with salt and pepper.
6. Pour the beans evenly on top, cover the pan again and cook over low heat for 20 minutes, or until the fish is opaque and firm when tested with a fork.

Summer Fruits Pudding

Serves 4–6

It is possible to make this all year round, using frozen berries.

Fat per portion is negligible.

225g (8 oz) raspberries
225g (8 oz) strawberries
115g (4 oz) wholemeal bread, sliced and
  crusts removed
120ml (4 fl oz) red grape juice
Suitable margarine for greasing

1. Wash the fruit.
2. Moisten the slices of bread with the grape juice.
3. Grease a pudding basin with a little margarine and line it with two-thirds of the bread slices, overlapping the edges slightly.
4. Put the berries into the basin and arrange the remaining slices of bread on top to cover the fruit.
5. Put a plate or saucer with weights on top and leave overnight in the refrigerator.
6. Remove from the refrigerator and lift off the weights and plate. Invert a serving dish over the top of the dish or basin and, holding the two firmly together, reverse them — giving a sharp shake. The pudding should slide out easily.

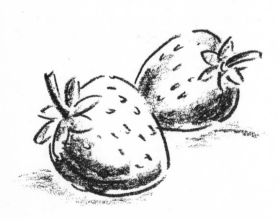

Friday

Orange juice
Wholegrain breakfast cereal
Skimmed milk
Dried or fresh fruit

Chilli con Carne (page 56)
Brown rice
Salad
Fruit salad, using fruit in natural juice

Sandwiches with mashed banana
Carob Brownies (page 57)
Fruit yogurt

Nutritional Information:

Fat (gms)	50
P/S ratio	2.0
Fat (%)	25
Fibre (gms)	45
Energy (Kcals)	1800

Chilli con Carne

Serves 6

Whenever you include mince in your diet, make sure it is lean mince or, better still, mince your own from any lean cut of beef. Vegetarians can substitute bulghur wheat for the minced beef.

Fat per portion = 20g

225g (½ lb) dried red kidney beans, soaked overnight in cold water
or
435g (15½ oz) tin red kidney beans
Salt
4 tablespoons corn oil
2 onions, peeled and chopped
2 garlic cloves, peeled and crushed
455g (1 lb) lean minced beef
1 green pepper, cored, seeded and chopped
1 teaspoon chilli powder
1 teaspoon paprika powder
1 teaspoon ground cumin
1 tablespoon tomato purée
1 tablespoon wholemeal flour
Freshly ground black pepper
2 × 395g (14 oz) tins tomatoes

1. Place the dried beans in a pan with a little salt and cover with cold water.
2. Bring to the boil, and boil vigorously for at least 10 minutes, then cover and simmer for 1 hour, or until tender.
3. Strain the cooking liquid and reserve 140ml (¼ pint). (If using tinned beans then drain and rinse under cold running water and reserve until needed.)
4. Heat the oil in a pan, add the onions and garlic and fry until golden.
5. Add the beef and green pepper and fry for 5 minutes, stirring constantly to break up the meat.
6. Stir in the chilli powder, paprika, cumin, tomato purée, flour and seasoning to taste and cook for 2 minutes.
7. Add the tomatoes and beans, stir thoroughly to mix, then bring to the boil.
8. Cover and simmer for 1-1¼ hours, stirring occasionally. If the mixture becomes too dry, stir in the reserved cooking liquid from the beans, or water if you used tinned beans.

Carob Brownies

Carob is said to be lower in fat than cocoa, and is an alternative to chocolate.

Fat per square = 13g

115g (4 oz) suitable margarine
115g (4 oz) sugar
2 eggs
55g (2 oz) wholemeal flour
30g (1 oz) carob powder
85g (3 oz) chopped walnuts

1. Cream together the margarine and sugar until light and fluffy.
2. Add the eggs to the mixture.
3. Sieve the flour and carob powder and add to the creamed mixture. Fold in the chopped walnuts.
4. Spoon into a lined 20cm (8-inch) square cake tin and bake in a pre-heated oven at 180°C (350°F/Gas Mark 4) for 30–35 minutes.
5. Remove from the tin and leave to cool. When cold cut into squares.

Saturday

Pineapple juice
Sliced apple and pear, topped with yogurt
   and honey
Wholemeal toast
Marmalade

Soused Herring (page 59)
Spinach Salad (page 60)
Wholemeal roll
Fruit crumble and custard (made with
   skimmed milk)

Chicken Liver Tagliatelle (page 61)
Salad
Fruit

Nutritional Information:

Fat (gms)	63
P/S ratio	1.7
Fat (%)	30
Fibre (gms)	35
Energy (Kcals)	1900

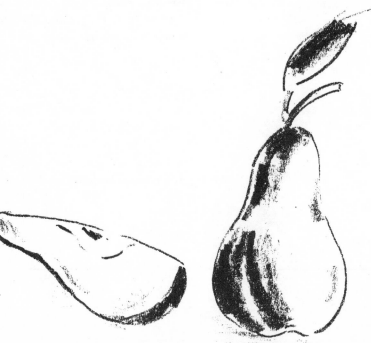

Soused Herring

Serves 6

Buy herrings that are as fresh as possible. If not available, choose frozen ones. Oily fish is a rich source of docosahexaenoic acid.

Fat per portion = 18g

6 herrings
1 onion, sliced
Vinegar
Water
4 bay leaves
2 cloves
12 allspice berries
2 mace blades
1 teaspoon salt

1. Preheat the oven to 300°F (150°C/Gas Mark 2). Clean the herrings and remove the fins, tails and backbones.
2. Lay the fish, skin down, on a working surface and place some sliced onion on the centre of each.
3. Roll the fish up from head to tail, secure with a wooden cocktail stick.
4. Place the fish in an ovenproof dish and add three parts vinegar to one part water to cover the fish. Add the herbs, spices and salt.
5. Cover and cook in the pre-heated oven for 3 hours, or until the fish is tender. The liquid must not boil.
6. Transfer the fish to a serving dish, strain the liquid over, cool, then chill in the refrigerator. The liquid sets into a soft jelly.

Spinach Salad

Serves 6

This refreshing salad is a traditional Iranian dish.

Fat per portion = 1g

850g (1 lb 14 oz) spinach
1 onion, chopped finely
1 teaspoon oil
2 cloves garlic, crushed
Salt and black pepper
225g (8 oz) natural yogurt

1. Trim the spinach. Wash, drain and shred coarsely.
2. Fry the onion in the oil, add the spinach and garlic, toss until wilted.
3. Cook until the moisture evaporates.
4. Remove from the heat, cool and season.
5. Pour the yogurt into a bowl, add the spinach mixture.
6. Toss well and adjust seasoning.

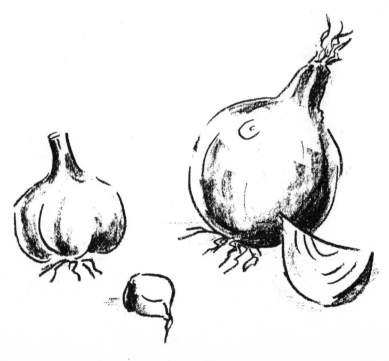

Chicken Liver Tagliatelle

Chicken livers are easily available, especially in frozen form, and are milder in flavour than other types of liver. The sauce in this recipe can be liquidized to give a smoother texture if this is preferred.

Fat per portion = 9g

2 tablespoons suitable oil
455g (1 lb) chicken livers, chopped
2 garlic cloves, crushed
395g (14 oz) tin tomatoes
½ teaspoon dried thyme
½ teaspoon dried basil
Black pepper
Salt
455g (1 lb) dried tagliatelle

1. Heat the oil over a moderate heat. Add the chicken livers and garlic and cook, stirring constantly, for 3–4 minutes or until the livers are lightly browned.
2. Add the tomatoes, thyme, basil and seasoning and bring the mixture to the boil, stirring.
3. Reduce the heat and simmer for 30–40 minutes, stirring occasionally.
4. Put the tagliatelle in a large saucepan of boiling water and cook until tender but still *al dente*. Drain, then pour over the sauce.
5. Using two large spoons, toss the mixture until it is blended. Serve immediately.

WEEK 3

Sunday

½ grapefruit
Baked beans on wholemeal toast

Roast chicken with Rice Stuffing (page 63)
Jacket potatoes
Broccoli
Roast parsnips
Gravy
Carob Pears (page 63) with fromage frais

Crunchy Salad (page 64)
Wholemeal roll
Nutty Apple Cake (page 65)

Nutritional Information:	
Fat (gms)	61
P/S ratio	1.7
Fat (%)	29
Fibre (gms)	51
Energy (Kcals)	1900

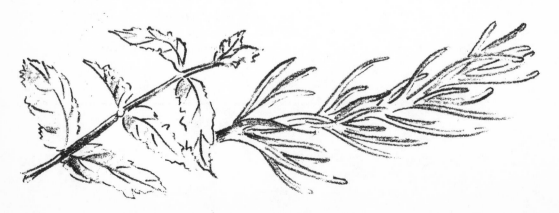

Rice Stuffing

This basic stuffing can be flavoured with herbs of one's choice, such as rosemary, cinnamon, basil, bay leaf or parsley. If the giblets came with the chicken, add the chicken liver to the stuffing mixture.

Fat per portion = 1g uncooked

55g (2 oz) short grain rice
1 medium onion, chopped finely
1 teaspoon suitable oil
Salt and pepper
900g (2 lb) chicken

1. Boil the rice until cooked. Drain, rinse and mix with the other ingredients, except the chicken.
2. Stuff chicken with the rice mixture.
3. Roast chicken in the usual way. When serving, reserve 455g (1 lb) of the meat for Monday (see page 67).

Carob Pears

Pears can be poached in a variety of liquids. Red grape juice imparts a red colour to the pears, and these look attractive served with natural yogurt.

Fat per portion = 3g

4 pears
1 teaspoon brown sugar
Juice 1 lemon
1 tablespoon grenadine (optional)
1 small bar of carob

1. Peel the pears, leaving stalks on.
2. Place in a pan of water with dissolved sugar and lemon juice plus grenadine if desired. Bring to boil and simmer gently for 15–20 minutes, or until pears are tender when pierced with a knife.
3. Melt the carob in a bowl over a pan of simmering water.
4. Take pears out of water and pour melted carob over top. Serve immediately.

Crunchy Salad

This salad makes a quick and easy addition to any lunch box, packed in a sealed container. Kept in the refrigerator it is also good for a quick snack.

Fat per portion = 3g

3 sticks celery
½ small cauliflower
2 crisp eating apples
Juice of 1 lemon
55g (2 oz) walnut pieces
225g (8 oz) skimmed milk soft cheese
½ teaspoon salt
Paprika pepper, to garnish

1. Wash the celery and cut into 2.5cm (1-inch) lengths.
2. Break the cauliflower into florets.
3. Quarter and core the apples. Cut into slices. Sprinkle with lemon juice.
4. Blend all the ingredients well together, except the paprika pepper.
5. Transfer to a salad bowl and sprinkle with the paprika.

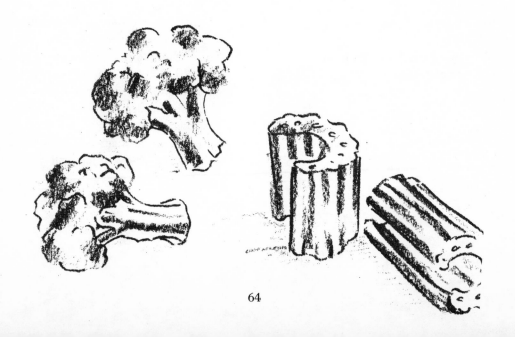

Nutty Apple Cake

The addition of a fruit such as apple or crushed pineapple makes a very moist fruit cake. This cake will keep for up to a week wrapped in foil, or in a cake tin.

Fat per slice = 16g

1 large cooking apple
28g (1 oz) walnuts
170g (6 oz) castor sugar
170g (6 oz) suitable margarine
225g (8 oz) self-raising wholemeal flour
1 teaspoon mixed spice
3 eggs
1 tablespoon skimmed milk
28g (1 oz) demerara sugar

1. Prepare a cool oven, 325°F (160°C/Gas Mark 3). Grease a round 18cm (7-inch) tin. Line base with greased greaseproof paper.
2. Peel and core the apple. Cut 6 thin slices and place in a bowl of cold water. Chop the remainder. Roughly chop the walnuts.
3. Place the sugar, margarine, flour, mixed spice, eggs and milk into a mixing bowl. Mix together with a wooden spoon, then beat for 2-3 minutes (or 1-2 minutes if using an electric mixer) until mixture is smooth and glossy.
4. Fold the chopped apple and walnuts into the cake mixture with a metal spoon. Place mixture in prepared tin, levelling the top with the back of the metal spoon. Drain remaining apple slices and arrange in a ring around the top of the cake. Sprinkle with demerara sugar.
5. Bake in the centre of the oven for 1¼-1½ hours. Test by pressing with the fingers; if cooked, the cake will spring back and will have begun to shrink from the side of the tin. Leave to cool in the tin for 15 minutes, turn out on to a wire rack and leave until cold.

Monday

Orange juice
Kipper
Wholemeal bread and margarine

Curried Chicken and Beansprouts (page 67)
Brown rice
Pineapple Sorbet (page 68)

2 egg omelette with spinach and fromage frais filling
4 Bean Salad (see Friday, Week 1, page 35)
Wholemeal roll
Fruit

Nutritional Information:

Fat (gms)	66
P/S ratio	1.5
Fat (%)	33
Fibre (gms)	31
Energy (Kcals)	1900

Curried Chicken and Beansprouts

Serves 3–4

Chicken is a very versatile meat and can be used in many ways. It is a lean meat and therefore suitable for including in your diet. Serve this recipe on a bed of brown rice.

Fat per portion = 7g

425ml (¾ pint) chicken stock
55g (2 oz) green pepper, chopped
55g (2 oz) celery, chopped
455g (1 lb) cooked chicken, cubed
  (from Sunday, lunchtime, see page 63)
225g (8 oz) beansprouts
1 teaspoon curry powder
Cornflour to thicken the sauce

1. Bring the stock to the boil.
2. Add the pepper and celery and simmer for 7–10 minutes until the vegetables are tender.
3. Add the chicken, beansprouts and curry powder and cook for a few minutes longer.
4. Thicken with the cornflour as necessary.

Pineapple Sorbet

This recipe needs to be made in advance.

Although fresh or frozen fruits are to be preferred, fruit tinned in natural juice is a useful store-cupboard item. It can be used in a variety of recipes, or on its own with fromage frais or natural yogurt.

Fat per portion is negligible.

225g (8 oz) unsweetened pineapple pieces

1 teaspoon lemon juice

1 small carton natural low-fat yogurt

1. Drain the pineapple and mix the juice and lemon juice into the yogurt.
2. Pour into a shallow container and freeze until the mixture is mushy.
3. Meanwhile, finely chop the pineapple.
4. Remove the mushy mixture from the freezer and mix in the chopped pineapple, beating thoroughly.
5. Return to the freezer and freeze until solid.
6. Transfer to the refrigerator an hour before serving.

Tuesday

Orange juice
Wholegrain breakfast cereal
Skimmed milk
Fresh fruit
Wholemeal toast with marmalade or jam

Tuna and Sweetcorn Savoury (page 70)
Jacket potato
Courgettes
Cabbage
Fruit and Nut Crumble (page 70) with
    custard (made with skimmed milk)

Pâté sandwiches
Side salad
Fresh fruit

Nutritional Information:

Fat (gms)	65
P/S ratio	2.2
Fat (%)	30
Fibre (gms)	41
Energy (Kcals)	1900

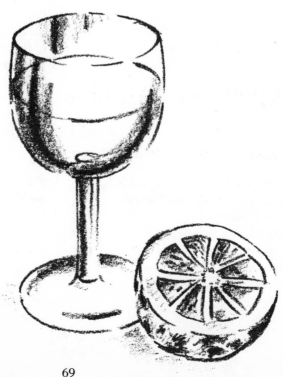

Tuna and Sweetcorn Savoury

Tinned fish should not be substituted for fresh or frozen fish in your diet, but tuna, sardines and pilchards are useful to have when fresh fish is not available. If tinned in oil, this should be drained off.

Fat per portion = 18g

1 onion, finely chopped
2 tablespoons suitable oil
200g (7 oz) tin sweetcorn, drained
200g (7 oz) tin tuna fish, drained
285ml (½ pint) skimmed milk
2 eggs
Salt and pepper

1. Fry the onion in the oil until transparent.
2. Put into the bottom of a 1 litre (2 pint) oven-proof serving dish.
3. Add the sweetcorn. Flake the tuna on to the sweetcorn.
4. Whisk together the milk and eggs and seasoning. Pour into the dish.
5. Cover with foil and stand in a roasting tin. Pour enough boiling water into the roasting tin to come halfway up the side of the dish. Cook at 350°F (180°C/Gas Mark 4) for 20 minutes.

Fruit and Nut Crumble

Sunflower and sesame seeds could also be added to this crumble mixture.

Fat per portion = 18g

455g (1 lb) prepared fruit (i.e., peeled, chopped and cored as necessary)
2 tablespoons water
55g (2 oz) suitable margarine
115g (4 oz) wholemeal flour
55g (2 oz) sugar
55g (2 oz) mixed nuts, chopped

1. Put the prepared fruit and water into a pie dish.
2. Rub the margarine into the flour until it resembles fine breadcrumbs.
3. Stir in the sugar and nuts and pour over the fruit.
4. Bake at 350°F (180°C/Gas Mark 4) for 45 minutes, until fruit is tender and topping brown.

Wednesday

Grapefruit segments
Poached egg on wholemeal toast (2 slices)

Poached smoked haddock
Boiled potatoes
Salad
Broccoli with sunflower seeds
Rhubarb and Honey Fool (page 72)

Lentil and Ham Soup (page 72)
Wholemeal bread
Fruit and yogurt

Nutritional Information:

Fat (gms)	52
P/S ratio	1.7
Fat (%)	27
Fibre (gms)	34
Energy (Kcals)	1800

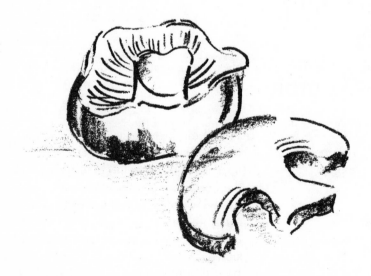

Rhubarb and Honey Fool

For a little extra luxury, decorate with small pieces of stem ginger.

Fat per portion is negligible.

455g (1 lb) rhubarb
2 tablespoons orange juice
2 tablespoons clear honey
140ml (¼ pint) yogurt

1. Trim the ends of the rhubarb and cut into 2.5cm (1-inch) pieces, removing any stringiness.
2. Place the rhubarb and the orange juice in a pan and simmer gently until the rhubarb is thoroughly cooked.
3. Stir in the honey and leave to cool.
4. Divide between 4 sundae glasses and swirl yogurt into each. Serve chilled.

Lentil and Ham Soup

Serves 4-6

Home-made stock gives soup a lot of flavour, but always make sure that you skim all the fat off the stock, especially with fatty meats such as ham.

Fat per portion = 5g

1 large onion, roughly chopped
4 large sticks celery, roughly chopped
2 large carrots, peeled and chopped
85g (3 oz) split yellow lentils
½ teaspoon dried parsley
Freshly ground black pepper
850ml (1½ pints) home-made ham stock
115g (4 oz) very lean, cooked diced ham

1. Put all the ingredients, except the ham, with 570ml (1 pint) of the stock in a large pan. Bring to the boil, then lower the heat, cover and simmer very gently for 1-1½ hours, or until everything is soft and mushy.
2. Purée in blender or work through a sieve.
3. Return to the pan.
4. Add the remaining stock and pieces of ham. Reheat gently.
5. Adjust seasoning and serve.

Thursday

Orange juice
Crunchy Muesli Mix (page 74)
Skimmed milk
Wholemeal toast
Sunflower seed spread

Beef and Orange Casserole (page 75)
Lyonnaise Potatoes (page 75)
Green cabbage
Braised celery
Tangy Bread and Butter Pudding (page 76)

Sandwiches filled with curd cheese and
    cucumber
Fruit and Nut Loaf (see Tuesday, Week 4,
    page 91)

Nutritional Information:

Fat (gms)	63
P/S ratio	1.6
Fat (%)	31
Fibre (gms)	33
Energy (Kcals)	1800

Crunchy Muesli Mix

By choosing a selection of ingredients from this recipe you can make your own muesli to suit your own tastes and preferences. Use not just as a breakfast cereal but also for a quick snack, or include in a variety of recipes from crumbles to crunch bars.

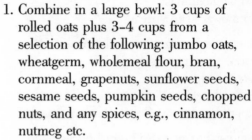

1. Combine in a large bowl: 3 cups of rolled oats plus 3–4 cups from a selection of the following: jumbo oats, wheatgerm, wholemeal flour, bran, cornmeal, grapenuts, sunflower seeds, sesame seeds, pumpkin seeds, chopped nuts, and any spices, e.g., cinnamon, nutmeg etc.
2. Combine separately, and pour over the dry ingredients, 1 cup of liquid made up from a selection of the following: honey, syrup, molasses, brown sugar, with 1 tablespoon of suitable peanut butter plus 1 tablespoon of suitable oil.
3. Bake in large greased baking pan at 300°F (150°C/Gas Mark 3) for 45 minutes, stirring often. The crunchiness can be varied, depending on proportions and cooking time. When cool, break into pieces and add raisins, dates, dried fruit or fresh fruit.

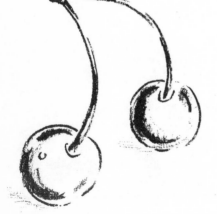

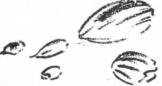

Beef and Orange Casserole

If you are a vegetarian, try substituting black eye beans instead of the beef in this recipe.

Fat per portion = 13g

680g (1½ lb) lean beef, cubed
Seasoned flour
1 large onion, sliced
1 clove garlic, crushed
3 tablespoons suitable oil
395g (14 oz) tin tomatoes
1 red pepper
3 sticks celery
140ml (¼ pint) orange juice
140ml (¼ pint) water

1. Toss the cubed beef in seasoned flour, then fry meat, sliced onion and crushed garlic in the hot oil.
2. Add the other ingredients, and cook, covered, in a moderate oven, 350°F (180°C/Gas Mark 4) for 2 hours.

Lyonnaise Potatoes

These can be cooked in the oven with the casserole.

Fat per portion = 13g

900g (2 lb) potatoes, peeled and thinly sliced
1 large onion, thinly sliced
55g (2 oz) suitable margarine
Salt and pepper
Chopped parsley

1. Blanch the potatoes in boiling water for 1 minute, then drain.
2. Fry the onion in the margarine until soft.
3. Layer the onion, potato and seasoning in a buttered 570ml (1-pint) casserole, finishing with a layer of potatoes.
4. Pour over any margarine left in the pan, cover and bake in a pre-heated oven at 400°F (200°C/Gas Mark 6) for 1 hour or, alternatively place on the top shelf in the oven with the casserole and bake for 2 hours at 350°F (180°C/Gas Mark 4).
5. Remove the lid for the last 30 minutes to allow the potatoes to brown. Sprinkle with parsley before serving.

Tangy Bread and Butter Pudding

The concentrated orange juice in this recipe gives a strong fruit flavour, making a change from traditional bread and butter puddings.

Fat per portion = 15g

8 slices bread spread with suitable margarine, crusts removed
55g (2 oz) sultanas
285ml (½ pint) skimmed milk
2 eggs
½ × 90ml (3 fl oz) tin concentrated orange juice, thawed
55g (2 oz) castor sugar

1. Cut the bread into squares. Layer, margarine side up, in a greased 1 litre (2-pint) dish, sprinkle with the sultanas.
2. Whisk lightly together the milk, eggs, orange juice and sugar. Pour over bread.
3. Place the dish in a roasting tin — half-filled with water. Cook at 375°F (190°C/Gas Mark 5) for 30 minutes, or until set.

Friday

Marinated Berries (page 78)
Wholemeal toast
Marmalade

Kidney Savoury (page 78)
Brown rice
Green beans
Carrots
Instant Cheesecake (page 79)

Lean meat salad
Wholemeal bread
Fruit

Nutritional Information:

Fat (gms)	57
P/S ratio	1.5
Fat (%)	28
Fibre (gms)	43
Energy (Kcals)	1900

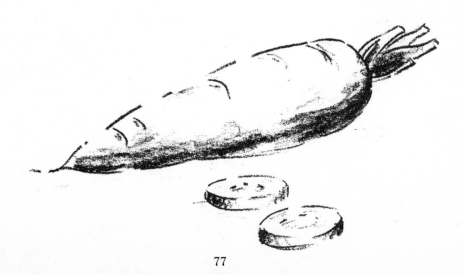

Marinated Berries

A sprinkle of chopped nuts can be added, but as nuts are high in fat, saturated and polyunsaturated, only small amounts should be used.

Fat per portion is negligible.

140ml (¼ pint) unsweetened orange juice
455g (1 lb) mixed berries, e.g.,
  raspberries, strawberries and
  blackberries
Yogurt, to serve

1. Pour the juice over the berries and leave to refrigerate overnight.
2. Serve with natural yogurt.

Kidney Savoury

Kidney, like liver, is an excellent source of vitamin B_{12} which is needed for the proper functioning of the nervous system. Eat kidneys as often as desired, but eat liver each week as well!

Fat per portion = 13g

6 kidneys
1 medium onion, chopped
115g (4 oz) mushrooms
28g (1 oz) suitable margarine
1 dessertspoon flour
Salt and pepper
2 tablespoons sherry
Chopped parsley, to decorate

1. Skin the kidneys, cut into slices and soak for an hour in salted water.
2. Gently fry the chopped onion, mushrooms and kidneys together in the margarine until tender.
3. Sprinkle with flour, add seasoning and gradually add the sherry.
4. Sprinkle with chopped parsley and serve straight away with boiled rice.

Instant Cheesecake

Serves 6

This cheesecake is so quick and easy, why make one any other way? This quantity will make 4 individual ramekin dishes so it can be served as individual portions. Useful when the biscuit base decides to be crumbly.

Fat per portion = 10g

115g (4 oz) crushed digestive biscuits
55g (2 oz) suitable margarine, melted
220g (7¾ oz) tin mandarins in natural juice, with the juice drained off
455g (1 lb) curd or preferably low-fat skimmed milk cheese
Vanilla essence

1. Mix the crushed biscuits with the melted margarine and press into an 18cm (7-inch) loose-bottomed cake tin or four individual ramekin dishes. Cool.
2. Mix the mandarins with the low-fat cheese, putting some aside for decoration. Add the vanilla essence.
3. Spoon on to the cold biscuit-crumb base and level.
4. Decorate with the remaining mandarins and chill in the refrigerator.

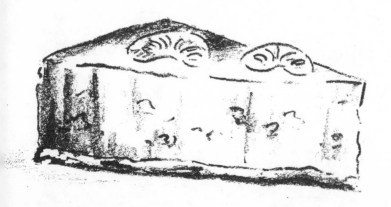

Saturday

Orange juice
Fried Plaintain (page 81)
Grilled mushrooms and tomato
Wholemeal bread

Shellfish Quiche (page 81)
Jacket potatoes
Salad
Apple and Cinnamon Pancakes (page 82)

Mediterranean Vegetable Soup (page 83)
Bread
Fruit

Nutritional Information:

Fat (gms)	48
P/S ratio	2.8
Fat (%)	27
Fibre (gms)	34
Energy (Kcals)	1600

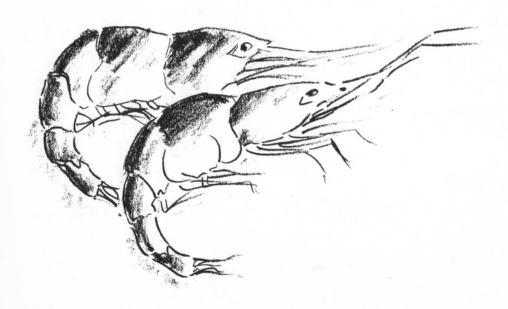

Fried Plantain

Fat per portion = 4g

2 medium-sized plantains (green bananas)
1 tablespoon suitable oil

1. Peel off the skin of the plantains and slice them thinly.
2. Fry in the oil.

Shellfish Quiche

Serves 6

Fat per portion = 16g

Pastry:

225g (8 oz) wholemeal self-raising flour
115g (4 oz) suitable margarine

4-6 spring onions
340g (12 oz) shellfish: include a variety from prawns, mussels, whelks, crab and shrimps
2 eggs
285ml (½ pint) skimmed milk
½ teaspoon tarragon

1. Make the pastry in the usual way and roll out to fit a 20cm (8-inch) flan dish.
2. Prepare and chop the onions.
3. Arrange the shellfish and onions in the pastry case.
4. Beat together the milk, eggs and tarragon, pour over the fish and onions.
5. Cook at 425°F (210°C/Gas Mark 5) for 20-40 minutes until the filling is set.

Apple and Cinnamon Pancakes

Makes 8

Pancakes are very versatile and can have savoury or sweet fillings. They are very easy to batch cook and freeze. Thaw from frozen in a hot oven.

Fat per pancake = 5g

Pancakes:

115g (4 oz) plain wholemeal flour
1 egg
285ml (½ pint) skimmed milk
Suitable oil for frying

Filling:

225g (8 oz) stewed apple
2 teaspoons cinnamon

1. Sift the flour and beat in the egg and skimmed milk.
2. Leave the batter to stand whilst seasoning the apple with the cinnamon.
3. Heat a small amount of oil in a frying pan and cook 8 pancakes, keeping the early pancakes warm until ready to use.
4. Divide the stewed apple mixture between the pancakes and roll them up.
5. Sprinkle with more cinnamon if desired.
6. Serve with natural fromage frais.

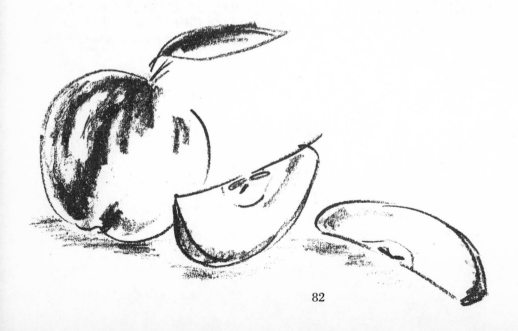

Mediterranean Vegetable Soup

Serves 6

Both the type and quantity of vegetables can be varied as desired.

Fat per portion = 5g

1 large potato
1 onion
115g (4 oz) carrots
115g (4 oz) frozen peas
55g (2 oz) celery
115g (4 oz) green beans
2 tablespoons suitable oil
215g (7½ oz) chopped tinned tomatoes
2 beef stock cubes dissolved in
  850ml (1½ pints) water
Dried herbs, as desired
Salt and pepper
Lemon juice (optional)

1. Clean and dice the vegetables.
2. Heat the oil in a large saucepan.
3. Add all the vegetables except the tomatoes and sauté for 10 minutes, stirring all the time.
4. Add the stock, chopped tomatoes, herbs and seasoning.
5. Bring to the boil, simmer for 1 hour, allowing the liquid to reduce for the last 20–30 minutes.
6. Season with lemon juice if desired.

WEEK 4

Sunday

Orange juice
Boiled egg
Wholemeal toast
Marmalade

Chinese Pork (page 85)
Brown rice
Green beans
Side salad and dressing
Fruit Fool with Sunflower Seeds (page 86)

Baked beans on wholemeal toast
Fruit
Yogurt

Nutritional Information:	
Fat (gms)	55
P/S ratio	1.2
Fat (%)	27
Fibre (gms)	43
Energy (Kcals)	1800

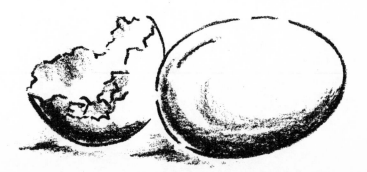

Chinese Pork

Serves 6

Very little preparation, but very tasty.

Fat per portion = 7g

1 onion, sliced
1 green pepper, chopped
1 tablespoon suitable oil
680g (1½ lb) very lean pork, cubed
225g (8 oz) tin pineapple cubes in
  natural juice, drained
140ml (¼ pint) natural pineapple juice
  (from the tin, make up with water if
  necessary)
3 tablespoons soya sauce
2 tablespoons soft brown sugar
2 tablespoons tomato purée
2 teaspoons made-up mustard
1 teaspoon ground ginger
Black pepper
Cornflour for thickening, if necessary

1. Fry the onion and green pepper in the
   oil. Add the pork.
2. Add all the other ingredients, except the
   cornflour. Stir well and bring to the boil.
3. Transfer to a casserole, cover and cook
   in the oven for 1 hour at 325°F
   (160°C/Gas Mark 3).
4. If required, thicken with some cornflour
   blended in a little cold water.

Fruit Fool with Sunflower Seeds

The fromage frais makes a very 'creamy' tasting fool and is a lot quicker and easier to use than making custard. Sunflower seeds are rich in linoleic acid, and can be added to a variety of recipes or nibbled as a snack.

Fat per portion is negligible.

225g (8 oz) fromage frais
455g (1 lb) stewed fruit, e.g.,
    gooseberries, rhubarb, etc
Sunflower seeds, as desired

1. Mix the fromage frais with the stewed fruit.
2. The sunflower seeds can be mixed into the fool whole, or can be liquidized to a fine powder and mixed in. Alternatively, they can just be used to decorate the top of the fool.
3. Chill in the refrigerator until required.

Monday

Grapefruit juice
Banana with natural yogurt, nuts and
    honey
Wholemeal toast
Marmalade

Lemon Mackerel (page 88)
New potatoes
Broccoli
Carrots
Fruit pie with custard or yogurt

Jacket potato with fromage frais and salad
Wholemeal roll
Fruit

Nutritional Information:

Fat (gms)	68
P/S ratio	1.9
Fat (%)	30
Fibre (gms)	45
Energy (Kcals)	2000

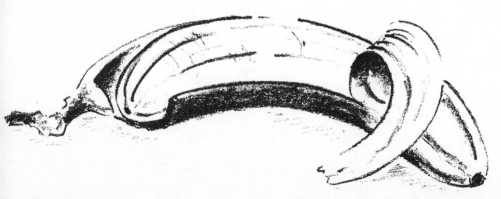

Lemon Mackerel

For special occasions, include some shellfish in the stuffing.

Fat per portion = 16g

Stuffing:

Suitable margarine for frying
1 small onion, finely chopped
85g (3 oz) fresh breadcrumbs
Finely grated rind and juice of 1 lemon
1 tablespoon chopped parsley
½ beaten egg

4 mackerel about 115g (4 oz) each, split and boned
Juice of ½ lemon
Salt and freshly ground black pepper
1 bay leaf, crushed
Water as required

1. Melt the margarine in a pan, add the onion and fry gently for 5 minutes or until golden.
2. Transfer to a mixing bowl and combine with remaining stuffing ingredients.
3. Lay the mackerel flat on a board and sprinkle the flesh with lemon juice and salt and pepper to taste.
4. Spoon the prepared stuffing into the fish and reshape.
5. Place in an ovenproof casserole, barely cover the bottom of the dish with water and add the bay leaf and more salt and pepper to taste.
6. Cover with a lid or foil and poach in a pre-heated oven at 325°F (160°C/Gas Mark 3) for 15–20 minutes, or until the fish is tender.
7. Drain and serve immediately.

Tuesday

Orange juice
Wholegrain breakfast cereal
Skimmed milk
Fresh fruit
Wholemeal toast and sunflower seed
    spread

Lentil Bolognese (page 90)
Spaghetti
Salad
Fruit salad
Fromage frais

Sandwiches filled with lean meat
Fruit and Nut Loaf (page 91)
Fruit

Nutritional Information:

Fat (gms)	38
P/S ratio	2.1
Fat (%)	21
Fibre (gms)	45
Energy (Kcals)	1700

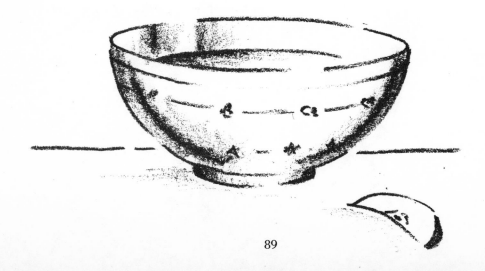

Lentil Bolognese

All kinds of pulses make lovely sauces for spaghetti. If you have a pressure cooker they can be cooked in a very short time. Split red lentils are particularly useful because they do not need to be soaked beforehand.

Fat per portion = 3g

225g (8 oz) split red lentils
1 onion, chopped
1 clove garlic, crushed
2 teaspoons suitable oil
115g (4 oz) mushrooms, sliced
1 green pepper, chopped
395g (14 oz) tin chopped tomatoes
2 tablespoons tomato purée
1 teaspoon oregano
Black pepper
225g (8 oz) wholewheat spaghetti
Parsley or watercress, for garnish

1. Wash the lentils. Put them in a saucepan, cover with cold water and simmer gently until they are cooked, about 25–30 minutes.
2. Fry the onion and garlic together in the oil for about 5 minutes, then add the mushrooms and green pepper and cook for a further 5 minutes or so.
3. Drain the lentils and stir them into the vegetable mixture, together with the tomatoes, tomato purée and seasoning.
4. Leave the mixture to simmer gently while you cook the spaghetti in boiling water until it is tender.
5. Serve the lentil sauce on top of the spaghetti on individual plates and garnish with parsley or watercress.

Fruit and Nut Loaf

This loaf contains no sugar, but gains sweetness from the dates and fruit it contains.

Fat per slice = 4g

140g (5 oz) wholemeal flour
2 teaspoons baking powder
1 teaspoon cinnamon
½ teaspoon mixed spice
28g (1 oz) suitable margarine
1 apple, grated
2 teaspoons grated orange rind
1 beaten egg
4 tablespoons skimmed milk
85g (3 oz) chopped dates or raisins
55g (2 oz) chopped walnuts

1. Sieve together the flour, baking powder, cinnamon and mixed spice. Cream the margarine with a little of the flour mixture.
2. Add the apple and orange rind, then the egg and milk.
3. Fold in the dates and nuts and the remainder of the flour mixture.
4. Bake in a greased 455g (1 lb) loaf tin at 325°F (170°C/Gas Mark 3) for 1 hour.

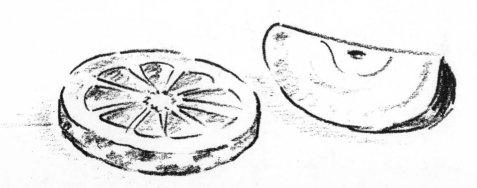

Wednesday

Orange juice
Baked beans on wholemeal toast
Fruit

Grilled haddock fillet, garnished with
    lemon and parsley
Jacket potato
Spinach
Sweetcorn
Eve's Pudding (page 93) and custard

Macaroni with Tomato Sauce (page 94)
Salad
Fruit

Nutritional Information:

Fat (gms)	36
P/S ratio	2.8
Fat (%)	18
Fibre (gms)	57
Energy (Kcals)	1900

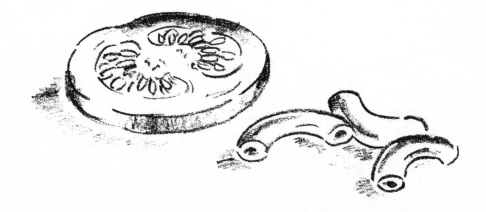

Eve's Pudding

As well as this fruit sponge, sponge sandwiches, cup cakes and gingerbreads can all be made by this simple method without creaming, so this basic recipe will be invaluable.

Fat per portion = 13g

455g (1 lb) stewed fruit
55g (2 oz) suitable margarine
55g (2 oz) castor sugar
115g (4 oz) golden syrup
1 egg
2 tablespoons milk
115g (4 oz) self-raising flour

1. Heat the oven to 375°F (190°C/Gas Mark 5).
2. Put the stewed fruit in an oven-proof casserole dish.
3. Put the margarine, sugar and syrup in a saucepan and heat gently until the margarine has melted.
4. Cool until lukewarm and mix in the egg and milk, using a wooden spoon. When well blended, add the flour and stir until quite smooth.
5. Spoon gently over the fruit and bake for 30–45 minutes, until golden brown.

Macaroni with Tomato Sauce

This tomato sauce freezes well. It can be made in large quantities and frozen. Re-heat from frozen slowly in a saucepan. This is an excellent vegetarian recipe.

Fat per portion = 9g

2 tablespoons suitable oil
2 onions, chopped
1 garlic clove, chopped
1 celery stalk, chopped
1 carrot, diced
2×395 (14 oz) tins chopped tomatoes
1 teaspoon dried oregano
1 bay leaf
570ml (1 pint) vegetable stock
2 tablespoons tomato purée
1 teaspoon Worcester sauce
Black pepper
340g (12 oz) wholewheat macaroni

1. Heat the oil and add the onions, garlic, celery and carrot. Allow to cook until soft.
2. Stir in the tomatoes.
3. Stir in the remaining ingredients, except the macaroni, and season.
4. Bring to the boil and simmer gently for 45 minutes. Liquidize if a smooth sauce is required.
5. Whilst the sauce is simmering, cook the macaroni in boiling water as directed. Pour the sauce over the cooked macaroni and serve.

Thursday

½ grapefruit
Scrambled egg and mushrooms
Wholemeal toast

Chicken Liver Risotto (page 96)
Three Pepper Salad (page 96)
Hot spiced fruit salad
Mock Cream (page 97)

Beetroot and Orange Soup (page 97)
Wholemeal roll
Cake (Fruit and Nut Loaf, see Tuesday,
   Week 4, page 91)
Fruit

Nutritional Information:

Fat (gms)	56
P/S ratio	2.4
Fat (%)	29
Fibre (gms)	37
Energy (Kcals)	1700

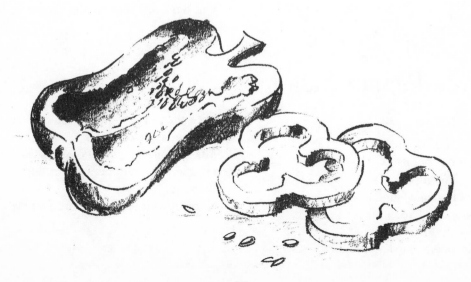

Chicken Liver Risotto

Fat per portion = 18g

1 onion, finely chopped
55g (2 oz) margarine
115g (4 oz) mushrooms, wiped clean and
  sliced
455g (1 lb) brown rice
570ml (1 pint) boiling chicken stock
8 chicken livers, cut into small pieces
2 tablespoons chopped fresh parsley

1. Fry the onion until soft in some of the margarine. Add the mushrooms and cook for a further 3 minutes.
2. Add the rice and cook, stirring constantly, for 2 minutes. Pour on the stock and let the rice cook over a high heat for 15 seconds.
3. Cover the frying pan, reduce the heat to low and simmer gently for 30–40 minutes or until the liquid is absorbed and the rice is tender.
4. While the rice is cooking, prepare the chicken livers: melt the remaining margarine, add the chicken livers and cook them for 10 minutes, stirring occasionally.
5. When the rice is cooked, stir in the chicken livers and parsley. Serve immediately.

Three Pepper Salad

Fat per portion = 8g

1 large yellow pepper
1 large red pepper
2 large green peppers
2–3 tablespoons sunflower oil
1 tablespoon lemon juice
Seasoning, to taste
2 tablespoons parsley, chopped

1. Slice the peppers thinly, making sure all the seeds are removed.
2. Mix the oil, lemon juice and seasoning together. Toss the peppers in the dressing.
3. Garnish with parsley before serving.

Mock Cream

A quick, low-fat cream substitute for serving with a variety of desserts, especially fresh fruit.

Fat per portion is negligible.

1 banana
1 tablespoon skimmed milk powder
1 egg white
4 drops vanilla essence

1. Mash the banana.
2. Add other ingredients and beat until stiff.

Beetroot and Orange Soup

This soup freezes well. Carrot can be substituted for the beetroot, to make a warming soup.

Fat per portion = 6g

28g (1 oz) suitable margarine
225g (8 oz) onion, finely chopped
Grated rind and juice of 1 orange
½ teaspoon cinnamon
2 cloves
1 bay leaf
995ml (1¾ pints) stock
455 (1 lb) beetroot, cooked and diced
Low-fat yogurt, to serve

1. Melt the margarine and fry the onion, orange rind, cinnamon, cloves and bay leaf until the onion is soft.
2. Remove the cloves and mix together the onion mixture, orange juice, stock and beetroot.
3. Bring to the boil and simmer for 20 minutes.
4. Remove the bay leaf, liquidize.
5. Serve with swirl of plain low-fat yogurt in each serving.

Friday

Pineapple juice
Crunchy Muesli Mix (see Thursday, Week
   3, page 74)
Skimmed milk
Wholemeal toast
Sesame seed spread

Sardine Loaf (page 99)
Mashed potato
Broccoli
Carrots
Fruit crumble and custard

Tabouleh (page 100)
Wholemeal roll
Fruit

Nutritional Information:

Fat (gms)	62
P/S ratio	2.0
Fat (%)	25
Fibre (gms)	52
Energy (Kcals)	2200

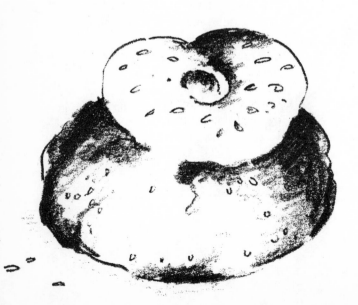

Sardine Loaf

Serves 6

An unusual recipe which makes a nice change from the traditional meat loaf. Tuna or pilchards can also be used in this recipe.

Fat per portion = 24g

115g (4 oz) suitable margarine
455g (1 lb) skimmed milk low-fat
  cheese
2×120g (4¼ oz) tins sardines, drained
2 cloves garlic, crushed
Juice of ½ lemon
Salt and pepper
Handful parsley, finely chopped
1 small loaf, wholemeal or granary, thinly
  sliced

1. Grease a 455g (1 lb) loaf tin.
2. Melt 85g (3 oz) of the margarine and cool slightly.
3. Mix the cheese and sardines together.
4. Stir in the garlic, lemon juice and melted margarine bit by bit.
5. Add the salt and pepper.
6. Mix together thoroughly.
7. Melt the remaining 28g (1 oz) margarine and stir in the chopped parsley, then spread the mixture on the base of the loaf tin.
8. Cut the rinds off the slices of bread.
9. Put a layer of bread on top of the parsley mixture, then a layer of sardine mixture, then bread, and so on, ending with a layer of bread.
10. Cover with a layer of foil and leave overnight in the fridge.
11. To turn out, dip the tin briefly in hot water and slip the loaf on to a serving dish. If necessary, smooth the sides with a knife. Keep in the fridge until needed.

Tabouleh

Serves 6

Fat per portion = 5g

115g (4 oz) cracked wheat (bulghur)
4 spring onions, finely chopped
2 tablespoons suitable oil
4 tomatoes, finely chopped (optional)
½ cucumber, finely diced
1 tablespoon mint (optional)
225g (8 oz) parsley
2 tablespoons lemon juice
Salt and black pepper

1. Soak the cracked wheat for 30 minutes in cold water.
2. Drain thoroughly and spread out on a plate to dry for a further 30 minutes, or squeeze with your hands.
3. Mix the spring onions with the cracked wheat and add the oil, tomatoes, cucumber, mint, parsley and lemon juice.
4. Season to taste and serve immediately.

Saturday

Apple juice
Porridge with dried fruit salad
Wholemeal toast
Marmalade

Chicken Casserole (page 102)
Jacket potato
Leeks
Cabbage
Grilled Bananas (page 102)
Yogurt

Home-made Pizza (page 103)
Salad
Fruit

Nutritional Information:

Fat (gms)	63
P/S ratio	1.9
Fat (%)	29
Fibre (gms)	64
Energy (Kcals)	1900

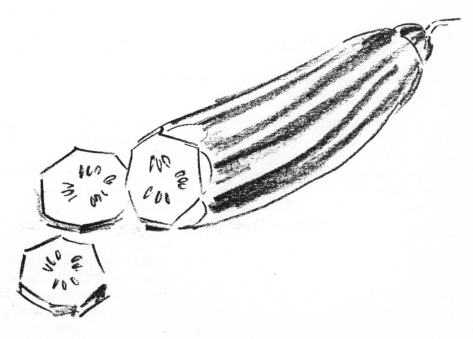

Chicken Casserole

It is important to remove the skin from the chicken, as the fat sits just underneath. Ready-basted chickens are not suitable for this dish or the EFA diet.

Fat per portion = 12g

4 chicken pieces, skin removed
2 tablespoons suitable oil
1 large onion, chopped
2 cloves garlic, crushed
115g (4 oz) mushrooms, sliced
1 green pepper, chopped
285ml (½ pint) chicken stock, plus 140ml
   (¼ pint) white wine
or
425ml (¾ pint) chicken stock

1. Brown the chicken pieces in the oil. Lift into a casserole dish.
2. Fry the onion and garlic until soft, then add the mushrooms and green pepper. Fry for 5 minutes.
3. Add the stock and wine (if used). Bring to the boil, then pour over the chicken.
4. Cook for 1–2 hours at 400°F (200°C/Gas Mark 4).

Grilled Bananas

A really quick dessert that is quite delicious. Serve with low-fat yogurt or fromage frais.

Fat per portion = 9g

Margarine for greasing
4 firm ripe bananas
Rind and juice of a large orange
Pinch each of ground nutmeg, cinnamon
   and cardamom
2 tablespoons honey or Barbados sugar
2 tablespoons flaked almonds, or sunflower
   seeds

1. Pre-heat a grill and brush a baking tray thinly with suitable margarine or vegetable oil.
2. Place the bananas, halved and split lengthways, on tray. Prick with fork 4 or 5 times.
3. Mix the orange juice, rind and spices in a cup, pour evenly over the bananas. Sprinkle with honey or sugar.
4. Grill for 3–4 minutes, sprinkle with almonds or sunflower seeds and grill for a minute or two more until they are golden.

Home-made Pizza

Pizzas do not always have to be covered in cheese to be moist and tasty. This recipe includes a very basic topping so experiment by using all sorts of vegetable and pulse purées as toppings. For an even quicker pizza, use this topping on French bread.

Fat per portion = 7.5g

Pizza base:

1 cup warm water
2 teaspoons dried yeast
1 teaspoon sugar
1 teaspoon salt
1 teaspoon oregano
150g (5¼ oz) wholemeal flour

Topping:

2 medium onions, cut into rings
1 clove garlic
1 tablespoon suitable oil
215g (7½ oz) tin tomatoes
2 tablespoons tomato purée
2 teaspoons oregano
Fresh tomatoes, sliced
50g (1¾ oz) tin anchovies

1. Put the warm water in a bowl and sprinkle on the dried yeast and sugar.
2. Add the salt and oregano.
3. Add sufficient wholemeal flour to make a soft but not sticky dough.
4. Cover and leave for 10 minutes.
5. Press into an 18×28cm (7×11 inch) oblong tin.
6. Fry the onions and garlic in the oil until soft.
7. Add the tomatoes, tomato purée and oregano and cook quickly to reduce the liquid and give a thicker consistency. Cook for 10–15 minutes.
8. Spread the topping over the pizza base and garnish with freshly sliced tomatoes and anchovies.
9. Bake in a pre-heated oven at 400°F (200°C/Gas Mark 6) for 25 minutes.
10. The top can be sprinkled with sunflower seeds or almonds before serving. These can be browned under the grill if desired.

MENUS FOR
DINNER PARTIES

Game Menu

Poached Monkfish with Cucumber and Dill

Casserole of Partridge with Savoy Cabbage
Mangetouts and baked potatoes

Bread and Butter Pudding with Sauce Anglaise

*This menu was put together by Roger, the
executive chef at Lilly's, a fish and game
restaurant in Clarendon Road, London W11*

Poached Monkfish with Cucumber and Dill

Fat per portion is negligible.

250g (9 oz) monkfish (or scallops), sliced
into finger-sized pieces
½ cucumber, cut into sticks
Juice of ½ lemon
1 bunch of dill

Vegetable stock:

680g (1½ lb) leeks
225g (8 oz) carrots
Bunch of parsley
Celery stick
1.7 litres (3 pints) water

1. Wash the vegetables to be used for the stock, then boil in the water for 30 minutes, or until reduced to 570ml (1 pint). Strain.
2. Shred the cooked carrots into strands.
3. Poach the monkfish (or scallops) and cucumber in the stock for 30 seconds, add the lemon juice and serve in deep plates, garnished with carrot strands and sprigs of dill.

Casserole of Partridge with Savoy Cabbage

All game birds and game meat are very low in fat, but rich in arachidonic acid. They are also becoming more readily available in supermarkets.

Fat per portion = 14g

1 Savoy cabbage
4 sticks celery
Chicken or pigeon bones (optional)
2 tablespoons tomato purée
2 tablespoons redcurrant jelly
2 teaspoons soya sauce
Partridges (allow one per person)
2 tablespoons suitable oil
Sprigs of parsley, for garnish

1. Cut up the Savoy cabbage, retaining the outer leaves.
2. Boil the celery, bones (if using) and the middle of the cabbage for 40 minutes, in 2.3 litres (4 pints) of water.
3. Strain and add the tomato purée, redcurrant jelly and soya sauce.
4. Poach the outer leaves of the cabbage in this mixture for 2 minutes, then cool, roll them up into round shapes and tie them.
5. Seal the partridges in a frying pan in suitable oil, then roast for 20 minutes. Allow to cool slightly then cut each partridge into four, placing the pieces in a casserole dish with the cabbage rolls. Cover with the stock.
6. Bake in the oven for 15–20 minutes. Untie the cabbage rolls before serving. The stock should by now have become a thick sauce.
7. Serve, garnished with sprigs of flat-leaf parsley and accompanied by mangetouts and jacket potatoes.

Bread and Butter Pudding

A 'nursery' pudding beloved by many people, but so simple to make.

Fat per portion = 5g

1 egg
75g (2¾ oz) fromage frais
75ml (⅛ pint) skimmed milk
Grated zest of 1 lemon
Thick sliced bread, spread with suitable
  margarine
50g (1¾ oz) currants
A little ground nutmeg

1. Whisk the egg until thick, then beat in the fromage frais, skimmed milk and lemon zest.
2. Line four ramekin dishes with sliced bread, scatter currants over each equally, then pour on the liquid and press down the bread. Sprinkle a little nutmeg on top of each.
3. Place the ramekins in a dish of hot water in the centre of the oven, cover them with foil and bake for 40 minutes at 350°F (180°C/Gas Mark 4), or until set.

Sauce Anglaise

Fat per portion = 2g

1 egg yolk
300ml (½ pint) skimmed milk
150g (5¼ oz) fromage frais
½ teaspoon vanilla essence

1. Whisk the egg yolk and milk together over a low heat until the mixture thickens. Remove from the heat. Beat in the fromage frais and vanilla essence.
2. Serve hot, with the Bread and Butter Pudding, which should be turned out.

Middle Eastern Menu

Baked Prawns

Liver Kebabs with Garlic

Potato Salad

Baked Courgettes

Strawberry Water Ice

Cinnamon or Aniseed Tea

Baked Prawns

Fat per portion = 9g

1 medium-sized onion, finely chopped
2 tablespoons polyunsatured oil
50g (1¾ oz) chopped spring onions
2 cloves garlic, crushed
170g (6 oz) peeled, chopped tomatoes
120ml (4 fl oz) dry white wine
8g (¼ oz) chopped parsley
½ teaspoon oregano
Salt
Freshly ground black pepper
400g (14 oz) peeled prawns

1. In a pan gently fry the onion in the oil until transparent, add the spring onions and garlic and cook for 2 minutes longer.
2. Add the tomatoes, wine, most of the parsley, oregano, and salt and pepper to taste. Cover and simmer gently for 30 minutes until thick.
3. Spoon half of the tomato sauce into 6 individual oven dishes or 1 large oven dish. Add prawns and spoon remaining sauce over them.
4. Cook in a very hot oven at 450°F (230°C/Gas Mark 8) for 10–12 minutes until prawns are heated.
5. Sprinkle with remaining parsley and serve immediately with crusty bread.

Liver Kebabs with Garlic

Fat per portion = 14g

400g (14 oz) lamb's liver
Cold salted water
3 cloves garlic
½ teaspoon dried mint
2 tablespoons suitable oil
Juice of 1 lemon
Salt
Freshly ground black pepper
Lemon wedges for serving.

1. Soak the liver in the water for 20 minutes. Drain, remove the skin from the liver and cut into 1cm (½-inch) slices. Cut the slices into roughly 2cm (¾-inch) squares. Dab the liver with paper towels to dry.

2. Crush the garlic and combine with the finely crumbled mint. Spread each side of the liver pieces with the garlic paste and place in a dish. Sprinkle with oil, lemon juice, salt and pepper to taste. Cover and leave for 30 minutes.

3. Thread pieces of liver on to skewers, passing them through the sides of the squares so that the liver is flat on the skewers.

4. Cook under a grill for a few minutes each side, taking care not to overcook. Brush with oil from the dish during cooking.

5. Serve hot with lemon wedges so that the juice may be squeezed over to individual taste.

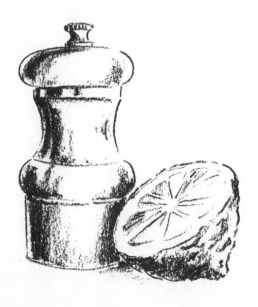

Potato Salad

Fat per portion = 8g

8 medium-sized potatoes
Salted water
1 medium-sized onion, finely chopped
15g (½ oz) finely chopped parsley
½ teaspoon dried mint
Salt
Freshly ground black pepper

Salad dressing:

1 clove garlic
1 teaspoon salt
Juice of 2 lemons
2 tablespoons polyunsaturated oil

1. Scrub the potatoes and boil in their jackets in salted water. When cool, cut into 2cm (¾-inch) cubes.
2. Place the potatoes in a bowl with the onion, parsley, mint rubbed to a powder and salt and pepper to taste.
3. Mix together the salad dressing ingredients and pour over the potatoes. Toss, and serve at room temperature.

Baked Courgettes

Fat per portion = 12g

400g (14 oz) courgettes
1 egg, beaten
3 tablespoons suitable oil
1 onion
400g (14 oz) tomatoes or 1 395g (14 oz)
    tin tomatoes
1 teaspoon brown sugar
Seasoning, to taste
1 teaspoon mint
1 tablespoon basil

1. Cut the courgettes lengthways and dip in beaten egg.
2. Gently fry in oil until the courgettes turn gold, drain on kitchen paper.
3. Chop the onion and fry for 5 minutes. Add the tomatoes, sugar and seasoning and cook for 20 minutes.
4. Place a layer of courgettes in a baking dish, then cover with sauce, sprinkle with mint and basil, then a layer of courgettes, and so on. Continue until all the ingredients have been used, ending with a layer of sauce.
5. Cover and bake in a pre-heated oven at 350°F (180°C/Gas Mark 4) for 20 minutes.

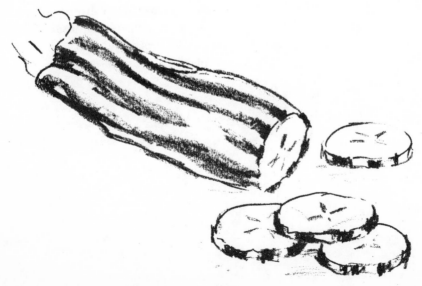

Strawberry Water Ice

Serves 6–8

Fat per portion is negligible.

Syrup:

450ml (16 fl oz) water
100g (4 oz) demerara sugar
2 teaspoons lemon juice

To finish:

340g (12 oz) strawberries
1 teaspoon strained lemon juice
60ml (2 fl oz) skimmed milk
Red natural food colouring

1. In a heavy pan combine the water and sugar and stir over heat until sugar is dissolved. Add the lemon juice and bring to the boil. Boil for 5 minutes, skimming when necessary, and leave until cool.
2. To make the strawberry purée, rub washed and hulled strawberries through a fine sieve. (This should yield 450ml/16 fl oz of purée.)
3. Combine the purée with the cooled syrup, lemon juice and milk and stir in a few drops of natural food colouring. Pour into a freezer tray or loaf cake pan and freeze.
4. Spoon into chilled dessert glasses and serve immediately. If desired, the ice can be broken up with a fork before placing in the glasses.

Cinnamon or Aniseed Tea

675ml (1¼ pints) water
4 large pieces of cinnamon
or
2 teaspoons cinnamon powder
or
2 teaspoons aniseed
75g (3 oz) finely chopped walnuts
   (optional)
Sugar, to taste

1. Put the water in a saucepan and add the cinnamon or aniseed.
2. Bring to the boil and boil gently for 5 minutes. If using cinnamon bark, remove it at the end of the boiling time. If using cinnamon powder or aniseed, strain the liquid.
3. Put a portion of nuts (if using) into each of 4 teacups. Pour the tea into the cup and add sugar to taste. Serve with a spoon if you have added the nuts.

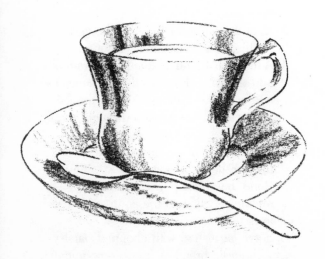

Italian Menu

Zuppe di Pesce (Fish Soup)

Pollo Arrosto (Roast Chicken with Rosemary)

Brown Rice

Green Salad

Orange and Kiwi Fruit Salad

Zuppe di Pesce (Italian Fish Soup)

Fat per portion = 11g

600g (1 lb 6 oz) whole fresh fish, e.g., red mullet
400g (14 oz) seafood, e.g., prawns, mussels, squid
2 tablespoons suitable oil
3 cloves garlic, crushed
1 red chilli pepper, seeded and chopped
1 large onion, chopped
1 stick celery, chopped
1 carrot, chopped
1 glass white wine
200g (7 oz) tinned tomatoes
Seasoning
Chopped parsley, for garnish

1. Clean the fish, keeping the heads to one side.
2. Clean and prepare the seafood if necessary.
3. Heat the oil and gently fry the garlic, chilli, onion, celery and carrot.
4. Add the fish and seafood and gradually add the wine. Finally add the tomatoes and continue cooking until all the fish and seafood are cooked through. (Squid, if included, will take longer.)
5. While the fish is being cooked, poach the fish heads in water for 20 minutes. Bone them and purée in a blender (optional). Stir into the soup, and season to taste.
6. Serve garnished with chopped parsley, with garlic bread as an accompaniment.

Pollo Arrosto (Roast Chicken with Rosemary)

Fat per portion = 14g

1.5kg (3 lb 5 oz) chicken
1 lemon, sliced
2 onions
1 clove garlic
1 tablespoon suitable oil
½ teaspoon rosemary
4 sage leaves
Seasoning

1. Stuff the chicken with sliced lemon and whole onions.
2. Crush the garlic and add with 1 tablespoon of the oil to the rosemary. Rub this mixture all over the chicken, and put the sage leaves under the wings and thighs. Season to taste.
3. Wrap in foil, put in a roasting dish and place in a pre-heated oven at 350°F (180°C/Gas Mark 4). Cook for 1½ hours.
4. Remove the foil, take out the stuffing, discard the lemon pieces and onions.
5. Make a gravy using the juices from the chicken.
6. Serve with brown rice and a green salad.

Orange and Kiwi Fruit Salad

Fat per portion = 2g

4 large oranges
2 kiwi fruits
1 tablespoon Cointreau
3 tablespoons orange juice
4 tablespoons Greek yogurt
1 teaspoon orange blossom water (optional)
1 tablespoon pine nuts

1. Peel and slice the fruit and arrange in individual dishes.
2. Mix the Cointreau and orange juice and pour over the fruit.
3. Top with 1 tablespoon of Greek yogurt flavoured with orange and orange blossom water, and a sprinkling of pine nuts.

Spanish Menu

Gazpacho (Iced Soup)

Paella

Apricot Soufflé

Gazpacho

Gazpacho is a refreshing soup on a warm evening, and is delicious with garlic or parsley bread.

Fat per portion = 5g

395g (14 oz) tomatoes
200g (7 oz) onions, chopped
1 teaspoon sugar
½ glass red wine
Salt and pepper
3 cloves garlic
2 teaspoons paprika
1½ tablespoons suitable oil
½ cucumber
10 black olives
Ice cubes, to serve
3 tablespoons parsley, chopped

1. Purée the tomatoes and mix with the chopped onion. Add the sugar, red wine and seasoning.
2. Mix the garlic, paprika and oil together and add gradually to the soup.
3. Dice the cucumber and add, together with the olives.
4. Cool in the fridge. Before serving, add ice cubes and chopped parsley.

Paella

Another traditional Spanish recipe, which is named after the dish in which it is cooked.

Fat per portion = 16g

400g (14 oz) mixed shellfish, including
  prawns, mussels, shrimps, clams
2 onions, chopped
1 red pepper, chopped
1 green pepper, chopped
3 tomatoes, chopped
2 cloves garlic, chopped
100g (3½ oz) chicken livers
3 tablespoons suitable oil, plus extra for
  frying
300g (10½ oz) brown rice
Salt
Saffron

1. Prepare the shellfish as necessary.
2. Fry the chopped onions, peppers,
   tomatoes, garlic and chicken livers in the
   oil, then add the shellfish and keep the
   mixture warm.
3. Using a large pan, heat 2 tablespoons of
   oil, add the rice, and stir until all the oil
   is absorbed.
4. Add 1 litre (1¾ pints) of boiling water,
   salt and saffron. Simmer until the rice is
   cooked, add the shellfish and tomato
   mixture and serve with Crunchy Salad
   (see page 64).

Apricot Soufflé

Fat per portion is negligible

100g (3½ oz) dried apricots
120g (4 fl oz) orange juice
4 egg whites, stiffly beaten

1. Stew the apricots in the orange juice and
   purée, using a blender, or put through a
   sieve.
2. Put into a greased, sugared soufflé dish.
   Fold in the stiffly beaten egg whites.
3. Bake in an oven preheated to 450°F
   (230°C/Gas Mark 8) for 15–20 minutes.

Oriental Menu

Sweetcorn and Crab Soup

Drunken Chicken with boiled rice

Celery Salad

Mango Sorbet

Sweetcorn and Crab Soup

Fat per portion is negligible.

1 teaspoon root ginger, chopped
2 teaspoons sherry
100g (3½ oz) crab meat
600ml (1 pint) stock
Salt
150g (5¼ oz) sweetcorn
1 teaspoon cornflour
1 egg white
1 spring onion, chopped

1. Mix the ginger, sherry and crab meat.
2. Heat the stock until boiling and add salt to taste, sweetcorn and the crab meat mixture.
3. When the mixture starts to boil, add the cornflour mixed with 2 teaspoons water, stirring constantly.
4. Add the egg white while stirring, and sprinkle the spring onion on top before serving.

Drunken Chicken

Fat per portion = 5g

1 young tender chicken
4 tablespoons dark soya sauce
120ml (4 fl oz) any Chinese wine or a pale
    sherry, not too dry
Spring onions, chopped unpeeled
    cucumbers, chopped fresh red chillies
    etc., for garnish

1. Lower the cleaned chicken into a
   saucepan of boiling water and simmer
   lightly for 30 minutes.
2. Drain the cooked chicken and place it
   whole in a bowl. Pour over it a mixture
   of the soya sauce and wine, and leave to
   marinate for several hours, spooning the
   juices all over the bird about every 30
   minutes.
3. When it is well soaked, carve the whole
   bird into pieces, arrange them nicely on
   a dish, pour over the marinade and
   garnish on top with the vegetables.
4. Serve with rice, which can be cooked in
   tomato juice to give an attractive colour.

Celery Salad

Fat per portion = 4g

4 sticks celery
2 green peppers
Salt
2 tablespoons soya sauce
1 tablespoon vinegar
1 tablespoon suitable oil
1 slice ginger root, finely chopped

1. Slice the celery and peppers and put in
   a pan of boiling salted water for 1 or 2
   minutes. Drain and rinse.
2. Mix together the soya sauce, vinegar and
   oil and add to the green pepper and
   celery. Toss well and garnish with finely
   chopped ginger root.

Mango Sorbet

If you do not have a food processor, then why not make an exotic fruit salad, using mangoes, lychees and mandarin oranges.

Fat per portion is negligible.

540g (1 lb 3 oz) tin mango pulp or 2
  fresh mangoes
300ml (½ pint) water
2 egg whites

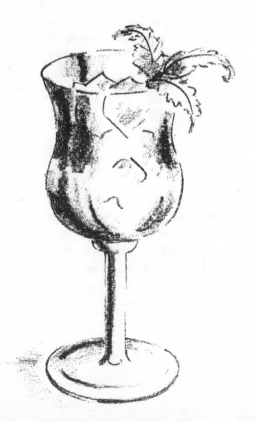

1. Prepare the mangoes if using fresh fruit. (Using a tin of mango pulp is far less fiddly than extracting the flesh from fresh mangoes.)
2. Mix together the mangoes and water in a food processor or liquidizer.
3. Freeze the mixture until it is half frozen.
4. Whisk the egg whites until stiff. Put the half frozen sorbet into the food processor, and when soft, gradually add the whisked egg white.
5. Refreeze the sorbet for 4 hours. Remove from the freezer 20 minutes before serving.

Dressings

3 tablespoons wine vinegar
6 tablespoons sunflower oil (or equivalent)
½ level teaspoon salt
¼ level teaspoon pepper
1 teaspoon French mustard

Put all ingredients into a screw-top jar or basin and shake or whisk together.

Variations:

Anchovy: Add 1 teaspoon anchovy essence.
Garlic: Add 1 clove garlic, crushed.
Lemon: Use lemon juice in place of wine vinegar.
Tarragon: Add 1 level tablespoon chopped tarragon.
Vinaigrette: Add 3 teaspoons chopped herbs.
Dill: Add 1 teaspoon fresh chopped dill.
Coriander: Add 1 teaspoon fresh chopped coriander.

INDEX

Of further interest

Multiple Sclerosis

A completely re-written edition of **Judy Graham's** much praised book, which includes the latest information on the links between MS and mercury in fillings, food allergies and saturated fats. It explains what MS *is*, self management techniques designed to prevent further deterioration, advice on food supplements, exercise, yoga and hyperbaric oxygen treatment. Also discusses mental and emotional factors, fatigue, relationships, sex, pregnancy and childbirth. Judy Graham has had MS for 12 years but by using the therapies in this book has succeeded in stabilizing her condition and continues to work as a freelance journalist in TV, radio and the press.

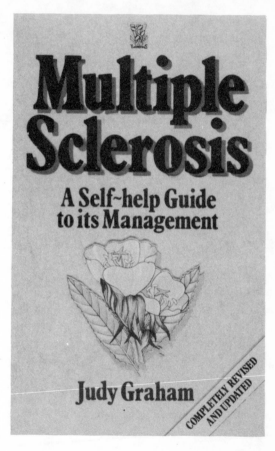